Seeking Strategic Advantage Through Health Policy Analysis

Beaufort B. Longest, Jr.

Health Administration Press
Chicago, IL 1996

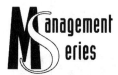

Management Series

Seeking Strategic Advantage Through Health Policy Analysis

01   00   99   98   97   5   4   3   2   1

Library of Congress Cataloging-in-Publication Data

Longest, Beaufort B.
    Seeking strategic advantage through health policy analysis /
Beaufort B. Longest.
        p.   cm.
    Includes bibliographical references and index.
    ISBN 1-56793-047-6
    1. Medical policy—United States—Evaluation.   2. Health planning—
United States.   I. Title.
RA399.A3L547   1996
362.1'0973—dc20   96-26898
                                                                        CIP

The paper used in this publication meets the minimum requirements of American National Standard for Information Sciences—Permanence of Paper for Printed Library Materials, ANSI Z39.48–1984.   ∞ ™

Health Administration Press
A division of the Foundation of the
   American College of Healthcare Executives
One North Franklin Street, Suite 1700
Chicago, IL 60606
312/424-2800

To the memory of my grandfather

Clemon Lazarus Faircloth

who taught me how to catch the elusive bluegill
and much about several of life's other wonderful secrets

Table of Contents

Preface

The ancient Chinese reserved a special curse for those they really disliked: May you live in interesting times. Someone must have placed this curse on the strategymakers in contemporary American healthcare organizations. If these are not interesting times for the people whose decisions guide this vast sector of the economy, it is difficult to imagine what they would find interesting. In fact, the times are more than—and worse than—merely interesting. In many ways, these are deeply troubled times in healthcare, so much so that the challenge of making appropriate strategic decisions for healthcare organizations is unprecedented.

The core strategic challenge for healthcare organizations remains unchanged. An organization's strategymakers still must decide what they wish their organization to be and to do, and how they want to go about accomplishing both. But these complex decisions are not made in a vacuum. The demands of the markets that an organization serves have much to do with its strategic decisions. So, too, do the actions and decisions of its competitors. And an organization's strategic decisions are heavily influenced by what goes on in its public policy environment.

This book is about the important link between public policymaking and strategymaking in healthcare organizations. This link is crucial, not only to healthcare organizations but also to the overall performance of the healthcare sector. This is reflected in the fact that this sector's most serious abiding problems, uneven access and cost inflation, are in large measure traceable to past failures or weaknesses in public policies. For example, policies that shape and guide the Medicare program provide extraordinarily generous benefits for the elderly and disabled, but without adequate cost containment provisions. Even more seriously, current policies do not provide adequate program funding for the future. Policies that guide the Medicaid program have never provided for the healthcare needs of all the poor, nor adequate funding for even the limited scope of the program. Policies that stimulate technological development have been formulated and implemented with little or no attention to healthcare technology's cost effectiveness or to its cumulative effect on overall healthcare costs. Policies that support the education of health professionals have helped produce a surplus of physicians and a serious imbalance between primary care and specialty care physicians. Still other policies have helped create grossly excessive hospital inpatient capacity.

Pointing out the shortcomings in these public healthcare policies is not to judge them as bad policies or to conclude that they should not have been enacted. Indeed, the Medicare and Medicaid programs are crucial to the millions of elderly, disabled, and poor Americans who rely upon government's ability to redistribute wealth as a means to offset the difficulties many people face in providing for their own needs. Which is worse, not enough hospital capacity or too much of it? Which would the nation prefer, limited medical technology or some that is not cost effective? Regarding most U.S. health policies, the issue is not whether the policies should exist at all; instead, the relevant issue is how to make the policies that are developed better. How can their beneficial aspects be enhanced and their weaknesses removed or minimized? In short, how can the public policymaking process, as it relates to healthcare, be improved?

One way to improve public policymaking for healthcare is by having the strategymakers in healthcare organizations take a more active and effective role in the public policymaking process. Their unique expertise and experience can be useful in this process. Beyond this, by playing a more influential role in the public policymaking process, strategymakers can improve the strategymaking that guides their organizations as well. In seeking to influence public policymaking to the strategic advantage of their organizations, strategymakers must learn more about the process. This knowledge can be used to better prepare their organizations to respond to the opportunities or defend against the threats inherent in particular public policies. In short, by becoming more involved in the public policymaking process, strategymakers can both improve the process and the policies that affect healthcare and at the same time enhance their own strategymaking.

This book's central premise is that strategymakers in healthcare organizations have two important and interrelated responsibilities regarding their organizations' public policy environments. They must both carefully *analyze* the public policy environments of their organizations, and they must seek to *influence* these environments to the strategic advantage of their organizations. This book is intended to show strategymakers how to carry out both responsibilities effectively.

Following the introductory chapter, Chapters 2 and 3, which are closely related, describe comprehensive conceptual models of the strategymaking and public policymaking processes. In combination, these models provide a context for the strategymakers in a healthcare organization to better understand their organization's external environment, including its public policy environment, and the relationships of this environment to strategymaking for the organization. Chapters 4, 5, and 6 then consider how the dual responsibilities of strategymakers to analyze and influence their organization's public policy environment can best be met. Chapter 7 provides a summary of the book's content through an applied example of the link between one organization's public policy environment and its successful strategymaking.

It is my hope that improved public policymaking for healthcare in the United States and improved strategymaking in the nation's healthcare organizations will help bring about the day when all our citizens receive healthcare that is fully appropriate to their needs. I further hope that improved policymaking and strategymaking will speed the day when all Americans receive their healthcare in seamless continua of care from organizations that consider improvement in the health status of those they serve to be their primary measure of success. If this book contributes in some small way to this future, even in one American community, then my time and energy in writing the book will have been well spent.

Beaufort B. Longest, Jr., Ph.D.
Pittsburgh, Pennsylvania
May 6, 1996

Acknowledgments

Some of the material on strategymaking contained in this book draws heavily on similar writing by the author in *Health Professionals in Management*, which was published by Appleton & Lange in 1996. Some of the material on the public policymaking process and on the public policy environments of healthcare organizations is adapted from *Health Policymaking in the United States*, which was published by Health Administration Press in 1994. Sincere appreciation is expressed to these publishers for permission to adapt and use this material in this book. I appreciate the contributions made by Professor Mark J. Kroll to the case study that appears in Chapter 7. It is an adaptation of his case, "University of Texas Health Center at Tyler."

I would like to thank the staff at Health Administration Press for their help and support in this project. I would also like to thank Carolyn Longest for her careful and constructive editing of this book's manuscript and Linda Kalcevic for her meticulous proofreading.

I would like to acknowledge my family for their patience with me during this time-consuming and, sometimes, all-consuming project. I thank my sons, Brant and Courtland, for all the pleasures of watching welcomed babies grow into exuberant and independent boys, and boys into fine young men. Most of all, I thank my beloved Carolyn who still makes many things possible in my life, and doing them seem worthwhile.

Introduction

The *strategies* of healthcare organizations are the sets of decisions that establish essential organizational characteristics such as ownership, interorganizational relationships, markets, and product lines. (Note that throughout this book, the term *organization* can mean an individual organization such as a hospital or it can mean an alliance or system of individual organizations. When the context does not make clear which is meant, specific labels are used.) Strategic decisions give organizations their positions and directions in relation to the overall external environments within which they exist. In effect, strategies are decisions about what an organization's leaders—or strategymakers— wish their organization to become and to achieve and how they wish to go about accomplishing this. Strategymaking, the process of making strategic decisions for an individual organization, or for a system or alliance of organizations, is the responsibility of senior-level managers, along with those who sit on governing boards. The strategymakers in healthcare organizations are the intended audience of this book.

Public Policies Strongly Influence Strategymaking in Healthcare Organizations

Many issues influence the strategies of healthcare organizations. Market forces are crucial influences on the strategymaking done for organizations that operate within market economies, such as the one in place in the United States. For example, the expressed preferences of buyers or purchasers of healthcare services in today's marketplace certainly drive much of the strategymaking that takes place in contemporary healthcare organizations. Their strategymakers seek constantly to find ways to satisfy the preferences of those who might purchase services in order to obtain and maintain marketshare. However, market forces are not the only concerns of strategymakers in healthcare organizations. They also seek to form and follow strategies that will permit their organizations to fulfill the missions established for them. Finally, and critically for the purpose of this book, public policies also play important roles in strategymaking for healthcare organizations.

Public policies are defined as authoritative decisions made in the legislative, executive, or judicial branches of government that are intended to direct or influence the actions, behaviors, or decisions of others. Numerous public policies pertain to or influence the pursuit of health in general and the strategies of healthcare organizations in particular, but strategymakers need to focus on more than the actual public policies. They must also concern themselves with the larger context within which these public policies are made. That is, they must also think about the intricate set of actors, actions, forces, and many other variables that make up the policymaking process itself. Only by thinking in this more expansive way can an organization's strategymakers focus effectively on its public policy environment.

Strategymakers who focus only on policy decisions after they have been reached, to the exclusion of the larger public policy environment in which those decisions are made, will be unprepared to make proper and timely strategic responses to policies as they emerge. Certainly, they will have had little if any influence in the intricate process through which the policies were established.

Public policies that pertain directly to healthcare organizations or that are strategically relevant to them constitute a very large set of decisions. Some of these decisions are codified in the statutory language of specific pieces of legislation. Others are the rules and regulations established to implement legislation or to operate government and its various programs. Still others are the relevant decisions made in the judicial branch. Thus, public policies may take any of several specific forms.

Whatever form public policies take, there are direct and powerful links between public policies, at both federal and state levels, and the strategic decisions that guide, shape, and direct healthcare organizations. In view of this strategically important relationship, the purpose of this book is to equip people who have, or who are preparing for, strategic responsibilities in healthcare organizations with a better understanding of the intricate relationships between public policies and strategymaking in these organizations. Along the way, the book also provides strategymakers with information about tools and perspectives that will permit their strategies to be more effective.

The Dual Responsibilities of Strategymakers Regarding Public Policy Environments

Much of this book's content is shaped by the fact that if strategymakers are to be successful they must fulfill two important and quite different responsibilities regarding their organizations' public policy environments.

First, effective strategymakers must be accurate in *analyzing* their organization's public policy environment. Such analyses include understanding the strategic consequences of events and forces in their organization's public policy environment. This means that they must be able to assess accurately the effects of public policies on their organizations, both in terms of opportunities and threats, and be able to position their organizations to make strategic adjustments that reflect planned responses to these effects.

Second, effective strategymakers must also be successful in *influencing* the formulation and implementation of public policies. Strategymakers have responsibilities to make their organization's environmental context, including the public policy component of that environment, as favorable as possible; failing that, they must make them as neutral to the organization as possible. Inherent in this responsibility is the requirement to identify public policy objectives that are consistent with their organization's values, missions, and strategic objectives and to help shape public policies accordingly through appropriate and ethical means.

The responsibility of strategymakers to analyze and influence policy is quite demanding. Even so, its importance to organizational performance requires that that responsibility be met. Consider for a moment, as an example, the extraordinary effects on the strategic decisions of many healthcare organizations inherent in policy changes, such as those listed below, that have been under consideration for the Medicare and Medicaid programs in recent years. Spurred by intense policy debates about the future of the Medicare and Medicaid programs, strategymakers throughout the healthcare industry have pondered such questions—with enormous potential strategic consequences for their organizations— as these:

- How would reductions in Medicare and Medicaid reimbursement rates affect our organization? How would such reductions change our strategies?

- What effects would increases in coinsurance payments on home health, skilled nursing care, and clinical lab services have on our organization? How would such changes affect our strategies?

- What proportions of the Medicaid and Medicare populations will be enrolled in managed care programs in the next few years? What would be the effects of such changes on our organization? How would these changes affect our strategies?

- How much and at what pace will inpatient use rates for our Medicaid and Medicare clients decline? What are the strategic implications of such declines?

- What policy changes is our state likely to make in view of efforts by the federal government to shift more of the costs of the Medicaid program to the states? How would our state's policy changes affect our strategies?

Obviously, questions such as these are very important to strategymakers facing anticipated Medicare and Medicaid policy changes. But these "consequence" questions reflect a serious strategic limitation: They typically arise *after* it is widely agreed that changes in policies will occur.

The ability to develop effective responses to the strategic consequences of policy changes is greatly enhanced when strategymakers are able to anticipate such changes months—or better still, years—ahead of when they actually occur. Beyond giving themselves the advantages of longer lead times to prepare for such changes, strategymakers who understand the inevitability of particular policy changes, even before the debate over the specific nature of the changes begins, can be positioned to influence emerging policies to the advantage of their organizations.

But how is such prescience to be achieved? By fulfilling the strategymaker's two fundamental and interrelated responsibilities: analysis and influence. Effective strategymakers foresee both the emergence and effect of relevant public policies on their organizations. This foresight enables them to begin to help shape the nature and scope of public policies that will affect their organization, often to its strategic advantage.

In fulfilling their dual responsibilities of analysis and influence, strategymakers must look beyond specific public policy decisions to the environments that created them. That is, strategymakers must focus not only on the policies that affect their organizations, but also on why and how these policies emerge. Strategymakers who focus broadly on their organizations' public policy environments increase their chances of anticipating policy changes far in advance of when those changes actually occur. This focus also influences the factors that lead, ultimately, to policies. It allows strategymakers actually to influence policies as they emerge. There is no doubt that strategymakers who understand the complex public policy environments from which the policies affecting their organizations emerge are better equipped both to anticipate and influence policymaking than their less-informed counterparts.

Equipped with a better understanding of the public policy environment that faces their organization, and endowed with a better comprehension of how their analysis and influence affects this environment, strategymakers would naturally consider a broader set of strategic questions than the "consequence" questions posed earlier. For example, strategymakers who were asking themselves "what if" questions about the dramatic change in the membership of Congress that took place after the 1994 elections, a shift heavily influenced by political promises to balance the federal budget and cut taxes, might well have predicted policy changes akin to those currently being made in regard to the Medicare and Medicaid programs. After all, there were and are only a very limited set of options available to deliver on both promises. Such questions as "What if the new Congress decides to use massive cuts in the Medicare and Medicaid programs as a means of helping achieve a balanced federal budget?" and "What if the federal government tries to change the Medicaid program into a block grant program as a means of stabilizing federal outlays for the program?" were being asked by some strategymakers in late 1994. By doing so, they gained a strategic advantage over their counterparts who waited until they were forced to ask the "consequence" questions about these developing changes.

There is always a vast difference between strategymaking based on solid predictions of future public policies versus strategymaking based on reacting to announced or soon-to-be-announced changes. With enough foreknowledge, proactive preparation and the opportunity to exert influence on the ultimate shape of policies are possible. If managers are caught by surprise after changes occur, only a reaction with inadequate time for a thoughtful response is possible.

"Consequence" questions, such as those suggested for Medicare and Medicaid policy changes, were indeed useful to guide reaction to the changes. But a different and far more valuable set of questions arose and were considered by the strategymakers who were carefully analyzing (and paying close enough attention to) the public policy environments that enabled them to envision changes far in advance of their occurrence and allowed them to influence those changes proactively. Strategymakers in healthcare organizations who pay close attention to their public policy environments reap the benefits of doing so.

Chapter Overview

Effective strategymaking in contemporary healthcare organizations is an extraordinary challenge. Not only are market forces and the moves of competitors affecting the strategies of these organizations more than ever before, but public policies continue to play crucial roles in their strategic decisions. If strategymakers in healthcare organizations are to be successful, they must simultaneously fulfill their dual analysis and influence responsibilities regarding the public policy environments of their organizations. Effective analysis in this context means to detect emerging policy changes as far in advance as possible and to consider what they will mean for the strategies of an organization. Effective influence means to help shape emerging policies that will affect an organization in ways that yield it some strategic advantage. The structure and content of this book are intended to provide strategymakers in healthcare organizations with the insights and tools needed to permit them to fulfill their analysis and influence responsibilities in relation to the public policy environments of their organizations.

This introductory chapter provides some key definitions to use throughout the book. Strategies, strategymaking, strategymakers, and public policies have been defined. The concept of an organization's public policy environment has been introduced, although much more will be said about this later. This chapter also emphasizes, as the book's central premise, that public policies strongly influence strategymaking in healthcare organizations, and it introduces analysis and influence, the two basic responsibilities of strategymakers regarding their organization's public policy environment. The following chapters are intended to equip strategymakers with both a better understanding of these responsibilities and with the tools and insights that will assist them in more effective strategymaking.

In Chapter 2: "Strategymaking in Healthcare Organizations," a framework is established for understanding the responsibilities of strategymakers to decide for entire organizations, or in some instances for alliances or systems of organizations that are purposefully linked together, what is to be done and how it is to be done. Strategic management is presented as a process of formulating and implementing organization-level strategies. A model of this process that incorporates four stages of activities is presented. The stages in the strategic management process are the conduct of situational analyses, including as part of this activity the analysis of an organization's public policy environment; strategy formulation; strategic implementation; and strategic control. The use of this model permits a consideration of how the responsibilities of strategymakers to analyze their public policy environments, along with their other external environments, fits into their larger responsibilities for the strategic management of their organizations.

In Chapter 3: "Public Policymaking," a model is used to show how public policymaking occurs in three interconnected phases: policy formulation, policy implementation, and policy modification. This model helps strategymakers understand the source of public policies as well as the nature and scope of the public policy environments they must analyze in carrying out their strategic responsibilities. This model is used later in Chapter 4 as a framework to help strategymakers know where to focus their analyses of public policy environments. Then, in Chapter 5, the policymaking model also becomes a framework for considering where within the policymaking process strategymakers can effectively intervene to influence public policies.

In Chapter 4: "Analyzing Public Policy Environments," the models of policymaking and strategymaking are integrated to help strategymakers better understand the relationships between these complex processes. A model of the standard process through which formal analyses of public policy environments are routinely conducted is presented. This model features environmental scanning to identify public policy issues of strategic importance; monitoring the strategic public policy issues identified; forecasting or projecting the future directions of strategic public policy issues; assessing the implications of the strategic issues for the organization; and diffusing the information obtained from its public policy environment within the organization so that the information can influence strategymaking.

In Chapter 5: "Influencing Public Policy Environments," the two most important pathways along which strategymakers can exert influence in their organization's public policy environment are considered. Following the first pathway, strategymakers can present and advocate their views and preferences, often through an association or interest group, and often in the form of lobbying, in an effort to have their views influence policies. Consideration is given to influencing public policies in this manner in the formulation, implementation, and modification phases of the policymaking process. The second important pathway, filing lawsuits in which policies or certain aspects of their implementation are challenged, is also presented. A background explanation of the political market for public policies is also given, which includes a consideration of those who demand and those who supply public policies that are related to healthcare organizations in the United States. Attention is also given to the ethics of influencing public policy, as well as to the roles of power and influence in the political marketplace.

Chapter 6: "Healthcare Interest Groups and Their Influence on Public Policy," builds upon the fact that the political economy of the United States features the collectivization of individuals and organizations with similar or related policy interests into interest groups for which the defining purpose is to serve the collective interests of their members. Interest groups seek to discern policy changes that might affect their members and to inform them about such changes. Thus, they can be of great help in carrying out the duties of strategymakers regarding the analysis of their public policy environment. Interest groups also seek to influence the formulation, implementation, and modification of policies for the purpose of providing the groups' members with advantages they might not otherwise enjoy. The capabilities of strategymakers in health-care organizations in both the areas of analyzing and influencing their public policy environments can be significantly enhanced by the activities of relevant interest groups. These opportunities for enhancement are described in this chapter.

Chapter 7: "An Applied Example: Strategymaking at the University of Texas Health Center at Tyler" contains a brief description of a real healthcare organization, along with an overview of its history. Then a series of questions about strategymaking in this organization are raised. In the answers that are provided for these questions, the key content of the book is summarized and applied in an actual strategymaking situation.

The book ends with Chapter 8: "Conclusion," in which the most essential points made in previous chapters are emphasized.

In the following chapter, the strategymaking process in healthcare organizations is examined in detail. In so doing, the management work through which strategymakers seek to both analyze and influence their organization's public policy environment to strategic advantage is de-scribed and considered.

Strategymaking in Healthcare Organizations

S trategymakers in healthcare organizations are the senior-level managers and members of governing boards who are responsible for making their organization's strategic decisions. These strategic decisions, or strategies, are the decisions that establish essential organizational characteristics, including ownership, interorganizational relationships, markets, and product lines. Strategies also give the organization for which they are developed their positions and directions in relation to their overall external environments. In effect, strategies are decisions about what an organization's leaders—or strategymakers—wish their organization to be and to achieve and how they wish to go about accomplishing this.

Although this book specifically focuses on the responsibilities of strategymakers for *analyzing* and *influencing* the public policy environments of their organizations, these dual responsibilities cannot be separated from the overall strategymaking process. Thus, this chapter describes the general strategymaking process in healthcare organizations in considerable detail.

The strategic responsibilities of an organization's senior leaders also extend to the implementation of strategies. When consideration of implementing strategies is added to the strategymaking process, the larger, more encompassing, process is thought of as strategic management. Both processes are modeled below.

A Model of the Strategic Management Process

There are four interrelated stages in the overall strategic management process as Figure 2.1 illustrates. The first two stages in this model, situational analysis and strategy formulation, constitute strategymaking (sometimes also called strategic planning). When the implementation and control stages are added, the entire process is thought of as strategic management.

Figure 2.1 Stages in the Strategic Management Process

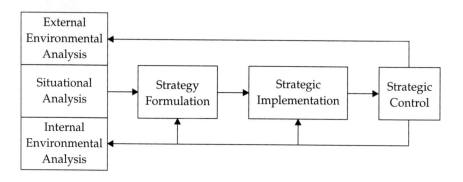

Source: *Health Professionals in Management* (p. 116), 1996 by B. B. Longest, Jr. Reprinted by permission of Appleton & Lange.

Each stage is considered in turn below. Remember, however, that the individual stages work together to accomplish strategic management.

Situational Analysis

The situational analysis stage of strategymaking has two components: external and internal environmental analyses. In this initial stage of the strategymaking process, strategymakers seek to identify and consider the opportunities and threats facing their organization from its external environment. In addition, they seek to identify and consider the internal strengths and weaknesses of their organization in the context of its philosophy and culture as well as its objectives.

External Environmental Analysis

The external environment for any organization includes all the factors outside its boundaries that can influence its organizational performance. It is useful to visualize the external environment of an organization, which is very complex, as shown in Figure 2.2. At the center of this conceptualization of an organization's external environment is the organization and the other similar, competing organizations. These form an industry; the hospital, nursing home, health maintenance organization, and pharmaceutical industries are examples.

The focal organization and the other organizations in its industry exist in a task environment. The task environment of an organization includes its industry and extends to clients or customers, suppliers, regulators, insurers, accrediting agencies, and so on with which the

Figure 2.2 The External Environment of a Healthcare Organization

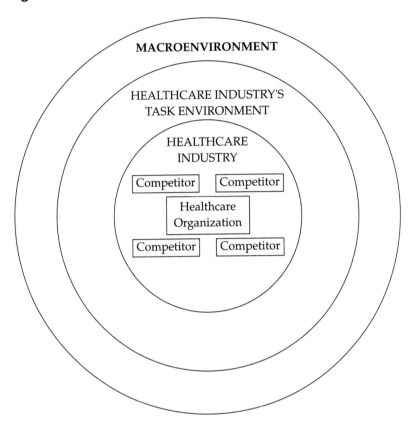

Source: *Health Professionals in Management* (p. 117), 1996 by B. B. Longest, Jr. Reprinted by permission of Appleton & Lange.

organization has direct interactions. Finally, the external environment of an organization includes its macroenvironment, or general environment, which comprises everything outside the industry's task environment.

In total, an organization's industry, task environment, and macroenvironment produce biological, cultural, demographic, ecological, economic, ethical, legal, policy, political, psychological, social, and technological information that the organization should include in its external environmental analysis. Public policies can be crucially important components of the external environments of healthcare organizations.

Healthcare organizations can be influenced, sometimes dramatically, by their external environments. In order to discern important information in their environments, strategymakers conduct formal external environmental analyses for their organizations. Although there are a number of approaches to conducting these analyses, they generally include five interrelated activities (Duncan, Ginter, and Swayne 1995):

- environmental scanning to identify strategic issues (i.e., trends, developments, opportunities, threats, or possible events) that could affect the organization;
- monitoring the strategic issues identified;
- forecasting or projecting the future directions of strategic issues;
- assessing the implications of the strategic issues for the organization; and
- diffusing the results of the analysis of public policy environments among those in the organization who can help formulate and implement the organization's strategies.

These five steps will form the basis for a detailed description and discussion of the process of analyzing public policy environments in Chapter 4.

Internal Environmental Analysis

The second step of the situational analysis stage of the strategic management process shown in Figure 2.1 is an internal environmental analysis. An effective and thorough internal environmental analysis includes a review of current strategy and a critical internal resource analysis in which both strengths and weaknesses inherent in the organization are identified and considered.

Current strategy is the set of decisions that determine the organization's essential characteristics and that give it position and direction in relation to its overall environment. A review of current strategy is conducted in order to establish a benchmark against which both strategy-making and strategic management take place. In effect, strategic managers review their current strategy to determine whether the organization is moving in the desired and appropriate direction, or whether some strategic changes are necessary. At the situational analysis stage, the review of current strategy is a rather perfunctory activity. It is not until the strategy formulation stage that this benchmark information is used to help determine if changes in strategy are to be made.

The internal resource analysis conducted in this stage is a straightforward process of cataloging the organization's internal strengths and weaknesses. This information can later be used to determine strategy by matching the organization's strengths and weaknesses against the opportunities and threats presented by the external environment. The order in which the external and internal analyses are made in the situational analysis is important because most internal strengths and weaknesses can only be identified in relation to the external environment. For example, a healthcare organization's "strong" financial position is defined in relation to the financial positions of other similar organizations. Similarly, an ambulatory surgery center's physical location is considered a strength only if there is ample demand for its services in the area in which it is located and if it enjoys a strong marketshare compared to its competitors.

The internal resource analysis (or audit) provides strategymakers with an inventory of their organization's resource base. The inventory should be compiled in a systematic manner. While there is no universal standard framework for conducting these inventories, a useful one includes the following components:

- a financial analysis covering the organization's financial condition, trends in its financial performance, and how it compares to industry norms;
- a human resources analysis covering the organization's capabilities in relation to its direct, support, and management work. This analysis should provide information on the adequacy of staff, in terms of numbers and quality, present activities, and possible future development;
- a marketing analysis covering all aspects of the organization's ability to distribute its services. This audit should identify the organization's markets and its competitive position (i.e., its marketshare) within these markets;
- an operations analysis covering the various production and service delivery activities of the organization. This analysis should cover activities in the direct work of the organization—for example, work done by the clinical departments and programs in a hospital—but it should also cover support and management operations as well; and
- an organizational culture analysis covering aspects of the shared beliefs (e.g., the centrality of patient care, the importance of medical research, the primacy of quality in healthcare services delivery) and values (e.g., duty, integrity, trust, and fairness) that help guide the behavior of all of the participants in an organization. While this analysis may involve a degree of subjectivity, it is nevertheless an important component of a complete internal resource analysis.

Strategy Formulation

The second stage in the strategic management process illustrated in Figure 2.1 is strategy formulation. Guided by the results of both the internal and external components of the situational analysis, strategymakers are positioned to establish organizational objectives, develop and evaluate strategic alternatives, select their strategy, and develop plans to implement it. This set of interrelated activities makes up the strategy formulation stage of the strategic management process.

The situational analysis in combination with strategy formulation constitute the strategymaking or strategic planning process in an organization. However, as will be seen below, strategymaking alone does not ensure that an organization's strategic objectives will be met. It only ensures their establishment. Strategic implementation and control must be added to strategymaking to complete the strategic management process as depicted in Figure 2.1.

Strategies can be formulated for three levels in organizations. Corporate-level strategies are developed for organizations formed into alliances or systems that operate as multiple units in multiple markets. A vertically integrated healthcare system with several acute care hospitals, a primary care center, a skilled nursing center, and a rehabilitation hospital would need such a strategy.

Corporate-level strategies should define the essential question of what businesses organizations are in. In seeking to define their businesses, strategymakers have strategic alternatives for changing the size as well as the scope and mix of products and services of their organizations. Duncan, Ginter, and Swayne (1992) categorize the possible corporate-level strategies available to organizations as either corporate growth strategies, which include diversification (related and unrelated) and vertical integration (forward and backward); or corporate degeneration strategies, which include divestiture and liquidation. See Table 2.1 for brief descriptions of these alternative corporate-level strategies. Of course, one possible corporate-level strategy is to remain the same, seeking neither growth nor degeneration.

Second-level strategies in organizations are called business-level strategies. Organizations that operate in single well-defined markets develop business-level strategies to address the question of how they should operate in their markets. Examples of such organizations include single-unit hospitals, nursing homes, group practices, and health maintenance organizations serving single markets. Organizations that are units of larger systems, systems that have corporate-level strategies, also develop business-level strategies. Business-level strategies for organizations that are units of larger systems are often called division-level strategies. No matter whether they pertain to single-unit organizations or to units of larger systems, or whether they are called business-level or division-level strategies, these strategies address the basic question of how the organization will operate in a given market.

Duncan, Ginter, and Swayne (1992) categorize the possible business- or division-level strategies available to organizations as business-level

Table 2.1   Corporate-level and Business-level Strategies

Corporate-level Strategies	Business-level Strategies
Growth	**Growth**
Related Diversification	*Market Share Building*
Entry into new markets with products and services that are similar to and synergistic with present products or services. This type of diversification is also called concentric diversification.	A functionally based strategy with the objective of growing (building relative market share) in present markets. Marketing usually plays a major role in market share building.
Unrelated Diversification	*Market Share Holding*
Entry into new markets with products and services that are unlike present products and services. This type of diversification is also called conglomerate diversification.	A functionally based strategy with the objective of maintaining relative marketshare within a market.
Backward Vertical Integration	*Turnaround*
Controlling the required inputs (raw materials, services, supplies, and so on) for present operations.	An aggressive functionally based growth strategy with the objective of reversing declining trends in market share, revenue, or profit.
Forward Vertical Integration	
Controlling the channel of distribution (delivery) for present operations or the flow of patients from one institution to another.	
Degeneration	**Degeneration**
Divestiture	*Market Share Harvesting*
Selling an operating business unit or division to another organization. Typically, the business unit will continue in operation.	Taking cash out and providing few new resources for a business in a declining market. Sometimes referred to as "milking" the organization.
Liquidation	*Retrenchment*
Selling all or part of the organization's assets (facilities, inventory, equipment, and so on) in order to obtain cash. These assets may be used by the purchasers in a variety of ways and businesses.	A decision to reduce the scope of operations, redefining the target market and selectively cutting personnel, products and services, or service area (geographic coverage).

Source: Adapted from Duncan, W. J., P. M. Ginter, and L. E. Swayne, *Strategic Management of Health Care Organizations*, p. 212. Boston: PWS-Kent Publishing Company, 1992; reprinted with permission.

growth strategies, which include marketshare building, marketshare holding, and turnaround strategies; and business-level degeneration strategies, which include marketshare harvesting and retrenchment strategies. These business-level strategies are also briefly described in Table 2.1.

The third level of strategies in organizations are the functional-level strategies, which are developed for the functional areas of organizations, especially in finance, marketing, human resources, and operations involving the direct work done in the organization such as that done by the clinical departments and programs in a hospital, as well as their support and management operations. Functional-level strategies are developed in single-unit organizations and in organizations that are units of larger systems. In effect, functional-level strategies represent the means through which business- and corporate-level strategies are implemented. For this reason, they are sometimes called implementation strategies.

No matter how carefully the corporate-, business- or divisional-, and functional-level strategies are developed for an organization, or how fully they reflect appropriate responses to the opportunities and threats identified in the situational analysis stage, an organization's strategies must be effectively implemented if the organization is to be successful.

Strategic Implementation

In the implementation stage of the strategic management process (see Figure 2.1), attention is turned to the challenges involved in carrying out strategies, challenges that can be very significant. Strategies, no matter how carefully crafted, do not implement themselves. Although related to strategymaking, strategic implementation is separate and distinct from it.

In the implementation stage, strategymakers blend their roles as strategists with their responsibilities for appropriately designing their organizations. That is, they rely upon carrying out their responsibilities for establishing patterns of relationships among people and other resources in their organizations as a means to help ensure that strategies are carried out. They also blend their roles as strategists with their responsibilities for motivating other people in the organization to achieve the organizational objectives established through strategymaking. Strategymakers invariably benefit by synergistically meeting their strategist, designer, and leader/motivator responsibilities (Longest 1996). Failure or inadequacy in any of these managerial responsibilities impairs the overall strategic management process.

A cardinal rule of good strategymaking is that strategymakers should not ignore implementation. There is a direct connection between an organization's capabilities to implement particular strategies and the appropriateness of such strategies for the organization. This connection is very important indeed. Organizations that are designed for implementing particular strategies are more likely to implement them well than organizations that have been designed for different strategies (Shortell,

Morrison, and Robbins 1985; Galbraith and Kazanjian 1986). For example, strategic managers in an organization that is designed for stability and centralized decisionmaking can have great difficulty in attempting to implement a corporate growth strategy of unrelated diversification. Similarly, people who are experienced only in implementing growth strategies will have difficulty shifting to degeneration strategies.

Ideally, an organization's strategic managers will recognize the connection between strategy and implementation capability in the formulation stage and factor this into strategic decisions. Sometimes, however, they do not. Degeneration strategies are often forced on organizations by the realities of their external environments, and in such cases, it does not matter that organizational participants prefer growth strategies. Consider what strategies have been forced on healthcare organizations by policies initiated to slow the rates of growth in the Medicare and Medicaid programs. In other cases, the preference of strategymakers for particular strategies overrides the fact that the organization's implementation capabilities are not well matched to the preferred strategies.

When mismatches occur between strategies and implementation capabilities, whether they are imposed by external policy or market changes or are the result of poor judgment on the part of strategymakers, problems invariably arise in the implementation stage of strategic management. Such mismatches can be overcome in two ways: (1) strategies can be changed; and (2) the capabilities of an organization to implement a strategy can be changed. In the latter case, resources can be redirected, people can be provided with additional training and education, and new people can be brought into the situation to support strategic implementation.

Even when there is a close match between strategies and implementation capabilities, strategic implementation requires that those with management responsibility for strategic implementation carry out their responsibilities in designing their organizations and in effective leadership and motivation. Their ability to design an appropriate organizational structure and to assemble a staff with the skills and abilities needed to carry out the implementation of strategies, including building and maintaining well-coordinated relationships among organizational units, are crucial factors in successful implementation. Similarly, the ability of strategic managers to motivate the necessary levels of effort on the part of many different organizational participants is vital to successful strategic implementation.

Strategic Control

The strategymaking and strategic management processes illustrated in Figure 2.1 are brought full cycle through a final stage, strategic control.

In this stage, strategic implementation is monitored, and the resulting information is used to control ongoing decisions, actions, and behaviors affected by the organization's strategies. Strategic control differs from operational control, which involves such activities as job, work, or production scheduling and statistical quality control, although both strategic and operational control follow the same basic paradigm that is outlined in Figure 2.3.

In the basic control process shown in Figure 2.3 actual results are monitored and compared to previously established objectives and standards, and deviations are corrected. In effective strategic control, strategymakers, who have overall responsibility for their organization's performance, evaluate that performance, and make changes when they are indicated.

Strategymakers must develop effective strategic control systems to support their efforts to achieve the successful implementation of their strategies by detecting discrepancies between desired and actual performance and by triggering corrective actions when necessary (Camillus 1986; Lorange, Morton, and Ghoshal 1986). Healthcare organizations typically employ a number of strategic control systems or devices, including budgets, routine activity reports, exception reports, employee

Figure 2.3 A Model of the Control Process

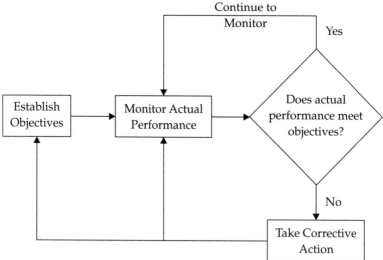

Source: *Health Professionals in Management* (p. 111), 1996 by B. B. Longest, Jr. Reprinted by permission of Appleton & Lange.

performance appraisal systems, and consumer or patient satisfaction surveys. Effective strategic control systems:

- facilitate coordination in organizations;
- motivate effort toward achievement of organizational objectives;
- provide an early detection system to warn that the assumptions and conditions underlying strategies are wrong or have changed; and
- provide a means through which strategymakers can intervene to correct an ineffective or inappropriate strategy.

Budgets are the most common strategic control system. They reflect projected activities of healthcare organizations, or units within them, in numerical terms covering a specified period of time. Their use as strategic control systems derives from their use as preestablished objectives or standards against which actual operating results can be compared and adjusted through the exercise of control. Budgets, like any good strategic control system, provide information that enables strategymakers to take corrective action when necessary to bring results into conformity with strategic plans. Although budgets often are expressed in monetary terms, they can be expressed in other units as well. Personnel budgets, for example, indicate the number of people needed at various skill levels and the number of working-hours allocated for certain activities.

Managers at all three organizational levels (first-, middle-, and senior-levels) participate in budgeting. The most effective approach, called "bottom-up" budgeting, has first- and middle-level managers prepare budgets for their domains, with senior-level managers (i.e., strategymakers) making adjustments to these when necessary and always giving final approval.

Budgets are merely guides for managers, not substitutes for good judgment. Effective budgets allow managers the necessary latitude and flexibility to accomplish the objectives established for their domains when conditions change within the period covered. To avoid having budgets become straitjackets, enlightened managers ensure flexibility in the use of budgets by monitoring operating conditions and revising established budgets when conditions appreciably change. The budgeting process is fairly complex, and its details are beyond the scope of this book. However, the reader will find useful guidance and insight into the process in such sources as Cleverly (1989) and Esmond (1990).

The Mechanisms of Strategic Control

Using Figure 2.3 as a guide, strategic control involves three steps: (1) establishing organizational objectives or strategies; (2) monitoring actual organizational performance; and (3) comparing it to performance objectives and correcting deviations.

Step 1: Establishing objectives or strategies. Strategies are established in the strategy formulation phase of the overall strategic management process. They are based on the results of the situational analysis that precedes formulation. As noted earlier in the discussion of strategy formulation, strategies are developed at three organizational levels—corporate, business or divisional, and functional. Strategy formulation for each level leads to the development of objectives for organizational performance at each level.

While some organizational objectives are inherently qualitative, others can be expressed in quite precise quantitative terms. Organizational mission statements, for example, tend to be qualitative. A children's hospital might list such qualitative objectives as these in its mission statement:

- provide comprehensive healthcare services to children that are appropriate to their special needs;
- advocate for the health and welfare of children;
- educate health professionals who will be involved in the care of children; and
- support research directed at obtaining a better understanding of the health problems of children.

In contrast to qualitative statements of organizational objectives, financial ratios such as return on investment, return on equity, debt to equity, and asset growth or such measures of market standing as overall marketshare or share of the target market, can be expressed with great quantitative specificity.

Step 2: Monitoring performance. In this second step of strategic control, strategymakers monitor actual performance in their domains and compare this to the desired states of performance they seek.

Where clear, concrete objectives and standards exist, monitoring outcomes and comparing them to the standards is a rather straightforward process. But to carry out this step effectively, strategymakers must observe more than mere operating results, although such bottom-line outcomes are always important in judging the success or failure of strategies. One very serious problem with relying on final outcomes is that they often occur too late to permit effective corrective actions necessary for fully meeting objectives. In addition to this problem, observation of final results may not point to why deviations occurred. To overcome such problems, effective strategymakers design their monitoring systems and techniques very carefully.

Management Information Systems (MIS) can be designed so that information relevant to strategic control can be collected, formatted, stored, and retrieved in a timely way to support the monitoring and comparing activities. These systems can be tailored to provide information that is useful in the strategic control of quality assessment and improvement as well as cost control activities, for example. If MIS are to be as useful as possible to support the monitoring and comparing of actual performance to desired standards of performance activities, they should possess certain characteristics, including:

- The MIS should match the elements of information it covers to the strategies being managed. The closer the match between the information and the specific nature and structure of strategies, the more effectively the strategic control step in the strategic management process can be carried out.

- The elements of information should indicate exceptions at critical points. Effective strategic control requires attention to those factors most critical to organizational performance. Generally, the more strategymakers concentrate their control efforts on critical points the more effective the results of their control efforts will be. Related to this characteristic, the elements of information in MIS should be economically selected. They should be worth their cost.

- The elements of information should be understandable to those who will use them. Some strategic control systems are supported by MIS, especially those based upon mathematical formulas, complex statistical analyses, and computer simulations, that include information elements that are not always understandable to the people who must use them. The inclusion of such elements in MIS can be dysfunctional.

- The MIS should report deviations promptly. The ideal MIS for strategic control purposes detects deviations soon after they actually occur. Only if information about difficulties with their strategies reaches strategymakers in a timely manner can they take effective corrective action.

- The MIS should be forward-looking. Although perfect control would be instantaneous, the facts of organizational life include a time lag between deviations and corrective actions in strategic management. Nevertheless, a crucial precursor to effective strategic control is the ability to detect potential or actual deviations from established strategies early enough to permit effective corrective action. Thus, strategymakers usually prefer a forecast of what will probably happen next month, next quarter, or next year (even though this contains a margin of error) to information, accurate to several decimal places, about events taking place in the past, about which nothing can be done.

- Finally, the MIS should point to corrective action. A strategic control system that detects deviations from established strategies will be little more than an interesting exercise if it does not lead to corrective action. An adequate system will disclose where failures are occurring and who is responsible for them, so that corrective action can be undertaken.

Step 3: Correcting deviations. In this step, corrective actions are taken to realign performance deviations with performance objectives. This step often presents difficult problems for strategymakers, even if they are guided by good information from their strategic control systems. It is often difficult to determine why strategies fail or why their implementation falters because so many underlying factors can be involved. One comprehensive model of such factors, known as the 7-S framework, has been developed by McKinsey & Company. This model's central premise is that seven variables (strategy, structure, systems, style, staff, shared values, and skills—the 7 S's) must all interact well with each other if strategy is to be successfully implemented (Waterman 1982).

The model of the strategic management process shown in Figure 2.1 illustrates that tracing the source or sources of deviations and deciding where to intervene to correct the underlying problems goes back to each stage of the process. Are the strategic assumptions that grew from the external and internal environmental analyses still valid? Are the strategies themselves still appropriate? Are the steps being taken to implement the strategies the correct ones?

Armed with a determination of the causes of deviations, strategy-makers can seek to take corrective action with some hope for a successful result. In this, strategymakers become agents of change. Thus, they are well served by remembering some of the key points in how people affect, and are affected by, organizational change:

- Any change process involves not only learning something new but also unlearning something that is well integrated into the personality and social relationships of the individual.
- No change will occur unless the motivation to change is present. Inducing that motivation is often the most difficult part of the change process.
- Organizational changes in authority structures, processes, and systems occur only through individual change by key members of organizations.

- Change involves altering attitudes, values, and behavior. The unlearning of present responses can initially be painful and threatening.
- Change is a multistage process, a complex cycle of behavioral modification that requires a systematic approach (Schein 1980, 243–44).

Strategic control, with its inherent organizational change, brings the strategic management process full cycle. This important step in the process is appropriately where strategymakers determine the continuing relevance of their strategies.

One of the important issues that the model of strategic management clearly illustrates is the relationship of public policies, developed in the external environments of healthcare organizations, to the strategies undertaken by these organizations. The importance of this intersection is explored in the next section as a prelude to examining a detailed model of the public policymaking process in Chapter 3.

The Intersection of Public Policymaking and Strategymaking in Healthcare Organizations

There is abundant evidence that the American healthcare system has been developed under extraordinarily favorable public policies. For example, the nation has long supported the development of medical technology through policies that directly support biomedical research and that encourage private investment in such research. For example, the National Institutes of Health (NIH) began in the early 1930s with annual budgets of about $10 million; today, their annual budget is approaching $12 billion. In addition, encouraged by public policies that permit firms to recoup their investments in research and development, private industry spends even more than the NIH on biomedical research and development.

Another important public policy that helped shape the contemporary healthcare system was enactment in 1946 of the Hospital Survey and Construction Act. Congress, in support of expanding availability of health services and improved facilities, enacted this legislation, known as the Hill-Burton Act, to provide funds for hospital construction. This marked the beginning of a decades-long program of extensive federal developmental subsidies to increase the availability of health services and facilities. To no one's surprise, the healthcare system has pursued a decades-long strategy of growth and expansion in physical facilities using the resources provided by this generous public policy.

Another important intersection between health policy and the strategic performance of healthcare organizations has been the expansion of health insurance coverage. Beginning during World War II when wages were frozen, health insurance and other benefits in lieu of wages became very attractive features of the American workplace. Encouraged by public policies that excluded these fringe benefits from income or Social Security taxes and by a Supreme Court ruling that employee benefits, including health insurance, could be legitimately included in the collective bargaining process, employer-provided health insurance benefits grew rapidly in the middle decades of the twentieth century (Health Insurance Association of America 1992).

In addition to private-sector growth in insurance coverage, Medicare and Medicaid legislation was passed in 1965, providing more access to mainstream medical care for the aged and many of the poor through publicly subsidized health insurance. With enactment of these programs, 85 percent of the American population had some form of health insurance.

Sustained and encouraged by these and other generous and supportive public policies, the healthcare industry in the United States has flourished. Following growth-oriented strategies, the U.S. healthcare system is by far the largest in the world. Furthermore, it has achieved unequaled levels of technical sophistication and excellence. Some of the major achievements of this industry include diagnostic and therapeutic capabilities that are the most advanced in the world, biomedical research that has brought scientists to the brink of understanding disease at the molecular level and intervening in diseases at the genetic level, and the availability of the latest technology and the most sophisticated clinical facilities to most Americans.

Whether public policies will continue to be as beneficial to the healthcare system, or as generous to the people the system serves, as they have over the past half-century is doubtful. The more draconian policies likely in the future could affect the strategic choices facing healthcare organizations even more dramatically than the supportive policies of past decades have. The important point is that both supportive and miserly public policies affect the strategymaking for healthcare organizations. The next chapter focuses on the complex process through which these public policies are formulated and implemented.

Summary

This chapter explores the process of strategic management in healthcare organizations. The first two stages of strategic management form the important process of strategymaking. Strategymaking, or strategic planning, is defined as deciding in advance for an entire organization what is to be done and how it is to be done. In strategymaking, organization-level objectives are established, and the means—plans or strategies—to achieve the objectives are formulated. The result of strategymaking is a set of plans or strategies to guide the organization, system, or alliance of organizations.

Strategic management describes the process of formulating and implementing organization-level strategies. A model of the four specific stages of the strategic management process has been presented. The stages, as shown in Figure 2.1, are situational analysis, which includes both an internal and external environmental analysis; strategy formulation; strategic implementation; and strategic control.

Strategic management involves managers at all organizational levels, although in different roles. Senior-level managers, along with their governing boards, formulate their organizations' strategies. But as a basis for doing this, they first conduct situational analyses, including assessments of internal strengths and weaknesses of the organization as well as the opportunities and threats presented to the organization by its external environment. And, in order to ensure that strategic implementation goes as planned, they must engage in strategic control. Middle- and first-level managers provide input to help guide formulation and participate in strategic control, but their primary responsibilities in strategic management are in strategic implementation.

Healthcare organizations are dynamic, open systems that exist in complex and turbulent external environments. They engage in ongoing exchanges with others in their external environments. This means that the organizations are affected, sometimes quite dramatically, by what goes on in their external environments. It also means that strategymakers in these organizations seek to influence their external environments. When managers acknowledge this reality, and when they permit their decisions and actions to reflect it, they are thinking and acting strategically. Two crucial elements in good strategic thought and action are effective analysis of the public policymaking environment faced by healthcare organizations to discern threats and opportunities, and effective influence on the public policymaking process. A model of this complex process will be presented in the next chapter as background for subsequent discussion of how strategymakers can best fulfill their responsibilities for both analyzing and influencing their public policy environments.

References

Camillus, J. C. 1986. *Strategic Planning and Management Control*. New York: Lexington Press.

Cleverly, W. O., ed. 1989. *Handbook of Health Care Accounting and Finance*, 2nd ed. Rockville, MD: Aspen Publishers, Inc.

Duncan, W. J., P. M. Ginter, and L. E. Swayne. 1992. *Strategic Management of Health Care Organizations*. Boston: PWS-Kent Publishing Company.

———. 1995. *Strategic Management of Health Care Organizations*, 2nd ed. Cambridge, MA: Blackwell Publishers.

Esmond, T. H., Jr. 1990. *Budgeting for Effective Hospital Resource Management*. Chicago: American Hospital Publishing, Inc.

Galbraith, J. R., and R. K. Kazanjian. 1986. *Strategy Implementation: Structure, Systems and Process*, 2nd ed. St. Paul, MN: West Publishing Co.

Health Insurance Association of America. 1992. *Source Book of Health Insurance Data*. Washington, DC: The Association.

Longest, B. B., Jr. 1996. *Health Professionals in Management*. Stamford, CT: Appleton & Lange.

Lorange, P., M. F. S. Morton, and S. Ghoshal. 1986. *Strategic Control*. St. Paul, MN: West Publishing Company.

Schein, E. H. 1980. *Organizational Psychology*, 3rd ed. Englewood Cliffs, NJ: Prentice Hall.

Shortell, S. M., E. M. Morrison, and S. Robbins. 1985. "Strategy Making in Health Care Organizations: A Framework and Agenda for Research." *Medical Care Review* 42 (Fall): 219–66.

Waterman, R. H. 1982. "The Seven Elements of Strategic Fit." *Journal of Business Strategy* 2 (Winter): 69–73.

Public Policymaking

As was emphasized in previous chapters, strategymakers in a healthcare organization have two very important sets of responsibilities regarding their organization's public policy environment. First, they are responsible for analyzing this environment. Done properly, this analysis permits them to understand the strategic consequences of events and forces in their organization's public policy environment. Such analysis yields an accurate assessment of the effects of public policies on the organization, both in terms of opportunities and threats. Furthermore, such analysis permits the strategymakers to plan responses to these opportunities and threats to their organization and to position themselves to make strategic adjustments.

Second, strategymakers are also responsible for influencing the formulation and implementation of public policies. This responsibility derives from the fact that effective strategymakers seek to make their organization's external environment, including the public policy component of that environment, as favorable to the organization as possible. Inherent in this responsibility are requirements to identify public policy objectives that are consistent with their organization's values, missions, and strategic objectives and to help shape public policies accordingly through appropriate and ethical means.

Fulfillment of both their analysis and influence responsibilities are demanding tasks for strategymakers. These responsibilities are made all the more demanding because healthcare organizations, perhaps as much or more than any organizations in American society, are affected by public policies. This fact stems from the fundamental contributions of healthcare organizations to the physical and psychological condition of the American people, as well as the role that these organizations play in the U.S. economy. In view of these very important contributions, it should not surprise anyone that government, at all levels, is keenly interested in the affairs of these organizations. This interest is reflected vividly in the attention that healthcare organizations receive within the expansive forum of public policymaking. This attention is translated directly into numerous public policies that pertain to or affect these organizations, including policies affecting the provision and financing of healthcare services as well as the production of inputs (e.g., the education of health professionals who work in the organizations and the development of technology that they use) to those services.

This chapter's central premise is that if strategymakers in healthcare organizations are to be effective at fulfilling their analysis and influence responsibilities in regard to the public policy environments of their organizations, they must fully understand and appreciate the complexity of the public policymaking process. This chapter is about this intricate process. An understanding of the process permits one to appreciate both the result of the process—the policies—and the context of the process—the public policy environment.

The chapter begins with some basic and underpinning definitions and concepts about the public policymaking process. Then, a general model of the process is presented. The model shows that policymaking includes three interconnected phases: policy formulation, policy implementation, and, eventually, policy modification. After the model of the public policymaking process is discussed, the outputs of the policymaking process, which are actual policies as well as perceptions about them and consequences of them, are shown to be important inputs to the strategymaking process in healthcare organizations.

Public Policy Defined

As defined in Chapter 1, public policies are authoritative decisions made in the legislative, executive, or judicial branches of government. A very important point about these decisions is that they are intended to direct or influence the actions, behaviors, or decisions of others. Some of these decisions are codified in the statutory language of specific pieces of legislation, while others are the rules and regulations established to implement legislation or to operate government and its various programs. Still others are the judicial branch's relevant decisions.

Public policies that pertain directly to healthcare organizations, or that are relevant to them, comprise a very large set of decisions. Examples include the establishment of the Medicare and Medicaid programs (P.L. 89–97), as well as subsequent amendments to this legislation; an executive order regarding operation of federally funded family planning clinics; a court's decision that the merger of two hospitals violated federal antitrust laws; a state government's decisions about its procedures for licensing healthcare organizations; a county health department's decisions about its procedures for inspecting the food services in healthcare organizations; and a city government's enactment of an ordinance banning smoking in public places within the city.

Indeed, the public policies that are of concern to strategymakers in healthcare organizations come in a variety of forms. For example, statutes or laws, such as the statutory language contained in the 1983 Amendments to the Social Security Act (P.L. 98–21) that authorized the prospective payment system for reimbursing hospitals for Medicare beneficiaries or the statutory language that defines which providers in a state can participate in the state's Medicaid program, are policies. Laws, when they are "more or less freestanding legislative enactments aimed to achieve specific objectives" (Brown 1992, 21), are sometimes called programs. The Medicare and Medicaid programs are examples. Another example on a smaller scale is the Special Supplemental Food Program for Women, Infants, and Children (WIC) program, which is a federal initiative undertaken to improve health by reducing nutritional deficits for the beneficiaries of the program. Still another example can be found in the Certificate of Need (CON) programs through which many states seek to influence capital expansion in their healthcare systems.

Another form that policies can take is that of rules or regulations established to implement laws and programs. Such rules, made in the executive branch of government by the organizations and agencies responsible for implementing laws and programs, and issued under the authority of law, are also policies. The rules associated with the implementation of complex statutes can fill thousands of pages. Rulemaking is an important component of the larger policymaking process modeled and discussed later in this chapter.

Judicial decisions are another form of policies. For example, the Supreme Court's reversal in 1988 of the earlier decision of the United States Court of Appeals for the Ninth Circuit in the *Patrick v. Burget* case (a case involving peer review of professional activities) is a policy by our earlier definition. This judicial decision is a policy because it is an authoritative decision that directs or influences the actions, behaviors, or decisions of others. As is often the case with judicial decisions, this one disrupted an established pattern of prior decisions and behaviors. Similarly, a decision issued in 1992 by a Department of Health and Human Services administrative law judge stated that a hospital was in violation of the Rehabilitation Act Amendments of 1974 (P.L. 93–516) when it prohibited an HIV-positive staff pharmacist from preparing intravenous solutions is also a policy (Lumsdon 1992).

Another form that public policies can take is so-called macro policies, a form only now emerging in the United States. Such broad policies "shape the health care system by constraining the flow of resources into it and setting limits on key players' freedom of action" (Brown 1992, 21). An example of such a policy would be the imposition by the federal government of a global budget for the nation's healthcare system. While macro policies are new to the United States, most other developed nations, notably Canada and Great Britain, have had such policies in place for their healthcare systems for decades.

Allocative vs. Regulatory Policies

The United States is a capitalist nation where presumably private markets best determine the production and consumption of products and services, including those produced by healthcare organizations. Although the volume and variety of existing public policies that affect healthcare organizations may seem incongruous with this fact, government generally intrudes with policies only when private markets fail to achieve desired public objectives. The most credible arguments for policy intervention in the nation's domestic activities begin with the identification of situations in which markets are not functioning properly.

The healthcare industry seems especially prone to situations in which private markets do not function well (U.S. Congressional Budget Office 1991). Theoretically perfect (i.e., freely competitive) markets, which do not exist in reality but provide a standard against which real markets can be assessed, require certain conditions:

- that buyers and sellers have sufficient information to make informed decisions;
- that a large number of buyers and sellers participate;
- that more sellers can easily enter the market;
- that each seller's products or services are satisfactory substitutes for those of their competitors; and
- that the quantity of products or services available in the market does not swing the balance of power toward either buyers or sellers.

The markets for healthcare services in the United States violate these underpinnings of competitive markets in a number of ways. The complexity of healthcare services reduces the ability of consumers to make informed decisions without guidance from the sellers or from other advisors. The entry of sellers in the markets for healthcare services is heavily regulated, and widespread insurance coverage affects the decisions of both buyers and sellers in these markets. These and other factors mean that the markets for healthcare services frequently do not function competitively, thus inviting policy intervention.

Furthermore, the potential for private markets, on their own, to fail to meet public objectives related to healthcare is not limited to the production and consumption of healthcare services. For example, markets might not stimulate the conduct of enough socially desirable medical research or the education of enough physicians or nurses without the stimulus of policies that subsidize certain costs. These and many other similar situations in which markets do not effect desired outcomes provide the philosophical basis for the establishment of public policies to correct problems. The nature of the problems they are intended to overcome or ameliorate help shape public policies in a direct way. Some problems require policies that regulate certain behaviors or actions if they are to be solved. Others may require changes in the allocation of society's resources. Public policies that are of interest to strategymakers in healthcare organizations fit broadly into allocative or regulatory categories, although there is considerable potential for overlap between the categories (Bice 1988; Williams and Torrens 1993).

Allocative Policies

Allocative policies are designed to provide net benefits to some distinct group or class of individuals or organizations, at the expense of others, in order to ensure that public objectives are met. Such policies are in essence subsidies through which policymakers seek to alter demand or supply of particular products and services, or to guarantee access to products and services for certain people. For example, on the basis that markets would undersupply the preparation of physicians without subsidies to medical schools, government has heavily subsidized the medical education system. Similarly, government subsidized the construction of hospitals for many years on the basis that markets would undersupply hospitals in sparsely populated regions or low-income areas.

Other subsidies have been used to ensure that certain people have access to healthcare services. The most obvious examples of such policies are the Medicare and Medicaid programs. In addition, state funding for mental institutions and federal funding to support healthcare for Native Americans, veterans, and migrant farm workers are other examples of allocative policies intended to assist individuals gain access to needed services. However, such subsidies as those inherent in much of the financial support for medical education, the Medicare program (the benefits of which are not based upon the financial need of the recipients) and the exclusion from taxable income of employer-provided health insurance benefits indicate that poverty is not a necessary condition for the receipt of the subsidies available in the allocative category of public policies.

Regulatory Policies

In a variety of ways, all levels of government seek to influence the actions, behaviors, and decisions of those who manage and work in healthcare organizations. As with allocative policies, government establishes regulatory policies to ensure that public objectives are met. There are five basic mechanisms of governmental regulation that directly affect healthcare organizations:

* market entry restrictions;
* rate or price-setting controls on healthcare providers;
* provider quality controls;
* market-preserving controls; and
* social regulation.

The first four of these are variations of economic regulation; the fifth seeks to achieve such socially desired ends as safe workplaces, nondiscriminatory provision of healthcare services, and reduction in the negative side effects that can be associated with the production or consumption of products and services (Bice 1988; Williams and Torrens 1993).

Regulations restricting market entry include those through which individual health professionals or healthcare organizations (e.g., hospitals and nursing homes) are licensed. Without a license, entry into a market is restricted. In addition to licensure regulations, state-operated CON programs require the state's approval for new capital projects by healthcare providers before the projects can be developed. Thus, they can restrict entry into markets. For example, a group of radiologists may be unable to obtain a CON for an ambulatory radiology center. Their entry into this market is precluded.

A common example of price regulation, another class of economic regulations, is government's control of the retail prices charged by public utilities such as those that sell natural gas or electricity. Although it is not classified as a public utility, the healthcare industry is also subject to certain price regulations. Several states have established hospital cost and rate-setting commissions. The federal government's control of the rates at which it reimburses hospitals for care provided to Medicare patients under the prospective payment system (PPS) of reimbursement and its establishment of a fee schedule for reimbursing physicians who care for Medicare patients are examples of rate regulation with enormous impact.

A third class of regulations are those intended to ensure that providers adhere to acceptable levels of quality in the healthcare services they provide and that producers of healthcare products such as imaging equipment and pharmaceuticals meet safety and efficacy standards. The federal government's Food and Drug Administration (FDA) is charged to ensure that new pharmaceuticals meet safety and efficacy standards. In addition, the Medical Device Amendment Act of 1976 places all medical devices under a comprehensive regulatory framework administered by the FDA. Another example of quality regulation can be seen in the federal government's establishment of an elaborate system of Professional Review Organizations, or PROs, to evaluate the quality and appropriateness of care rendered to Medicare beneficiaries.

Because the markets for healthcare services do not behave in truly competitive ways, government intervenes in these markets by establishing and enforcing rules of conduct for market participants. These rules form a fourth class of regulation, market-preserving controls. Antitrust laws, such as Sherman Antitrust Act, the Clayton Act, and the Robinson-Patman Act, which are intended to maintain conditions that permit markets to work well and fairly, are a good example of this type of regulation.

Importantly, the United States is entering a new era in regard to market-preserving regulations in the healthcare industry as it moves toward managed care as the basic structure of the industry. Managed care stimulates the development of integrated networks of healthcare services providers that can compete with each other for groups of insured people within a framework that encourages cost-conscious decision making by consumers (Coddington, Moore, and Fischer 1996; Shortell et al. 1996). If managed care is to work well, it will likely require the elaboration of new market-preserving regulations. For example, regulations pertaining to the inclusion of publicly-sponsored Medicare and Medicaid beneficiaries in managed care systems have already become necessary.

The four classes of regulations outlined above are all variations of economic regulation. The primary purpose of social regulation, the fifth class of regulation, is to achieve such socially desirable outcomes as workplace safety and fair employment practices and to reduce such socially undesirable outcomes as environmental pollution or the spread of sexually transmitted diseases. Social regulation usually has economic effect, but the effect is secondary to the primary purposes of this category of regulations. Federal and state laws pertaining to environmental protection, disposal of medical wastes, childhood immunization requirements, and the mandatory reporting of communicable diseases are but a few obvious examples of social regulations that affect healthcare organizations.

Whether public policies take the form of statutes or laws, programs, rules and regulations, judicial decisions, or macro policies, they are always established within the context of a complex public policymaking process. Both allocative and regulatory policies are made within that process, and the activities and mechanisms used to create both categories of policies are essentially identical. A comprehensive model of this process that can apply to any level of government is described later in this chapter. But first it will be useful to consider certain aspects of the political market for public policies.

The Marketplace for Public Policies

An understanding of the marketplace for public policies, the so-called political market, is largely based on a knowledge of the operation of traditional economic markets. Economic markets and political markets share a number of common features. Many kinds of products and services, including those used in the pursuit of health, are bought and sold in the context of economic markets. In these markets, willing buyers and willing sellers enter into economic exchanges involving something of value to both parties. One party demands and the other supplies. By dealing with each other through market transactions, individuals and organizations buy needed resources and sell their outputs. Political markets operate in much the same way, at least conceptually. However, there are certainly some key differences.

The most fundamental difference between economic and political markets is that in economic markets consumers express their preferences by spending their own money. That is, in economic markets consumers reap the benefits and directly bear the costs of their choices. In political markets, on the other hand, the link between who receives benefits and who bears costs is not as direct. These markets differ in other ways as well.

> In private markets individuals make separate decisions on each item they purchase. They do not have to choose between sets of purchases, such as between one package that may include a particular brand of car, a certain size house in a particular neighborhood, several suits, and a certain quantity of food. Yet in political markets their choices are between two sets of votes by competing legislators on a wide variety of issues. While individual voters may agree or disagree on parts of the package, they cannot register a vote on each issue, as they do in economic markets.
>
> Voting participation rates differ by age group. The young and future generations do not vote, and yet policies are enacted that impose costs on them. Future generations depend on current generations and voters to protect their interests. However, as has been the case many times, such as with respect to the federal deficit and Social Security, their interests have been sacrificed to current voters.

Legislators use different decision criteria from those used in the private sector. A firm or an individual making an investment considers both the benefits and the costs of that investment. Even though a project may offer very large benefits, profitability cannot be established unless its costs are also considered. Legislators, however, have a different time horizon, which not only affects the emphasis they place on costs and benefits but also on when each is incurred. Since members of the House of Representatives run for reelection every two years, they are likely to favor programs that provide immediate benefits (presumably just before the election) while delaying the costs until after the election or years later. Further, from the legislator's perspective, the program does not even have to meet the criterion that the benefits exceed its costs, only that the immediate benefits exceed any immediate costs. Future legislators can worry about future costs (Feldstein 1988, 237–38).

Public policies are among the commodities valued in the political marketplace (Marmor and Christianson 1982). Both those who "supply" policies and those who "demand" or "consume" policies recognize their innate value; in political markets, both suppliers and demanders stand to reap benefits or incur costs because of policies. In order to understand the policymaking process, one must first appreciate the interplay between the demand and supply sides of the marketplace for public policies.

Because policies can be made in the executive, legislative, and judicial branches of government, the list of potential suppliers of public policies—the policymakers—is lengthy. Members of each branch of government play roles as suppliers of policies in the political market, although the roles are played in very different ways, as will be seen more clearly in Chapter 5. The potential demanders of public policies also constitute a lengthy list. Obviously, this list includes healthcare organizations whose strategies are influenced in any way by public policies.

Thinking of political markets as operating similarly to economic markets—that is, as markets in which something of value is exchanged between suppliers and demanders—permits public policies to be viewed as valued commodities, as a means of satisfying certain demanders' wants and needs in much the same way that private products and services serve to satisfy demanders (usually called consumers) in private economic markets. In private markets, demanders seek products and services that satisfy them. In political markets, demanders specifically seek public policies that satisfy their preferences.

The contemporary marketplace for health policies is a lively place indeed: a place where many participants seek to further their objectives. These objectives can be self-interest objectives, perhaps involving some economic advantage, or public-interest objectives involving certain participants' perception of what is best for the nation. In both cases, the outcome depends greatly on the relative abilities of participants in the exchanges within the marketplace to influence actions, behaviors, and decisions of other participants.

The discussion of how the suppliers and demanders of public policies interact in the political markets for these policies provides a background for considering the intricate process through which policies are made. As will be seen, the motivations and behaviors of the participants in this process follow closely those outlined above. This makes the process more understandable and predictable, although in playing out this process in the real world there are always a few surprises.

The Public Policymaking Process

As Figure 3.1 illustrates, the public policymaking process is distinctly cyclical. The circular flow of the relationships among the various components of the model is one of its most important features. Policymaking is a continuous process in which almost all decisions are subject to subsequent modification.

Another important general feature shown in the model is that the entire policymaking process is influenced by factors that are external to the process. This makes the process an open system—one in which the process interacts with its external environment. This is shown by the impact of biological, cultural, demographic, ecological, economic, ethical, legal, psychological, social, and technological inputs on the process.

One feature that the model does not show is the political nature of the process in operation. This is important to recognize if the complexity of the policymaking process is to be fully appreciated. The process would be simpler, and perhaps better, if it were driven exclusively by fully informed consideration of the best ways for policy to serve the public interest, by open and honest debate about such policies, and by the rational selection from among policy choices strictly on the basis of ability to contribute to the pursuit of health. Those who are familiar with the policymaking process, however, know that it is not driven exclusively by these considerations. A wide range of other intervening considerations influence the public policymaking process. The preferences and influence of interest groups, political bargaining and vote trading, and ideological biases are among the most important of these other factors. Truth and rationality do indeed play parts in health policymaking. On a good day, they will gain a place among the flurry of political considerations. But, as has been noted, "it must be a very good and rare day indeed when policy makers take their cues mainly from scientific knowledge about the state of the world they hope to change or protect" (Brown 1991, 20).

Figure 3.1 A Model of the Public Policymaking Process in the United States

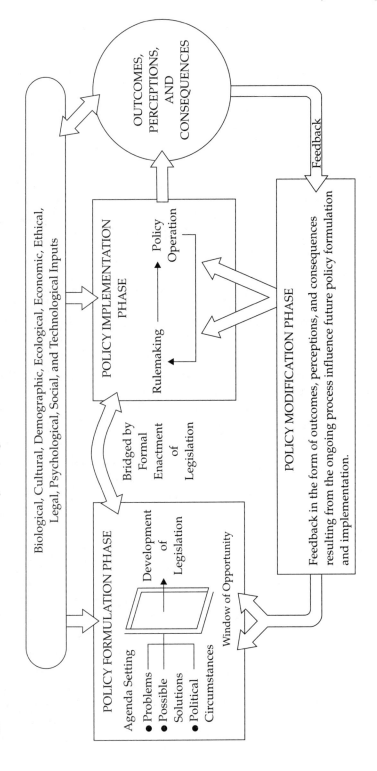

Source: *Health Policymaking in the United States* (p. 32), 1994 by B. B. Longest, Jr. Adapted by permission of AUPHA/Health Administration Press.

The public policymaking process includes three interconnected phases:

- policy formulation, which incorporates activities associated with agenda setting and subsequently with the development of legislation;
- policy implementation, which incorporates activities associated with rulemaking and policy operation; and
- policy modification, which allows for all prior decisions made in the process to be changed.

The formulation phase (making the decisions that lead to legislation) and the implementation phase (taking actions and making additional decisions necessary to implement legislation) are bridged by the formal enactment of legislation, which shifts the cycle from its formulation to implementation phases.

Policies, once enacted as laws, still need to be implemented. This responsibility rests mostly with the executive branch, which includes many departments (e.g., the Department of Health and Human Services and the Department of Justice). It also includes the activities of a number of independent federal agencies such as the Consumer Product Safety Commission and the Federal Trade Commission (FTC). These departments and agencies in the executive branch of government exist to implement the policies embodied in legislation.

It is important to remember that some of the decisions made within the implementing organizations, as they put policies into effect, become policies themselves. For example, rules and regulations promulgated in order to implement a law are policies just as are the laws whose implementation the rules support, as was discussed earlier in this chapter. Similarly, judicial decisions regarding the applicability of laws to specific situations or the appropriateness of the actions of implementing organizations are decisions that are themselves public policies.

The policy modification phase exists because perfection cannot be achieved in the other phases and because policies are established and exist in a dynamic world. Suitable policies made today may become inadequate with future biological, cultural, demographic, ecological, economic, ethical, legal, psychological, social, and technological changes.

Policy modification, which is shown as a feedback loop in Figure 3.1, might entail nothing more than minor adjustments made in the implementation phase or modest amendments to existing legislation. In some circumstances, however, the outcomes and consequences of implementing certain policies can lead all the way back to the agenda-setting stage of the process. For example, the challenge of formulating policies to contain healthcare costs facing policymakers today is, to a large extent, an outgrowth of the success of previous policies that expanded access and subsidized an increased supply of human resources and advanced technologies to be used in the provision of healthcare services.

One should keep in mind, as the separate components of this policymaking model are examined individually and in greater detail in subsequent sections, that the model depicts a political process, a process that is cyclical in its operation, a process that is heavily influenced by factors external to the process, and a process whose component parts are highly interactive and interdependent.

The Policy Formulation Phase

The formulation phase of the policymaking process includes two distinct and sequentially related sets of activities: agenda setting and legislation development (see Figure 3.1). The nation's health policies comprise a myriad of decisions that emerge from a diverse array of problems, possible solutions to the problems, and dynamic political circumstances. At any point, there are many problems or issues related to health. Many of them have possible solutions; often they have alternative solutions, each of which can have its supporters and its detractors. The existence of problems and potential solutions is overlaid by diverse political interests. The ways in which particular issues emerge from this mix to advance to the next stage in the policymaking process is an important feature of the process and is termed "agenda setting" in the model.

Once health policy issues rise to prominent places on the political agenda, they can, but do not always, proceed to the next stage of the policy formulation phase, which is labeled "Development of Legislation" in the model. At this stage, specific legislative proposals go through a process involving a carefully prescribed set of steps that can, but do not always, lead to policies in the form of new laws or statutes or, as is more often the case, amendments to previously enacted statutes. Only a small fraction of the potential universe of policy issues emerge from the agenda-setting activity in the right circumstances that provide the impetus for them to reach the point of having specific legislation developed to address the issues. And, even then, only some of the attempts to enact legislation are successful. The path for legislation can be long and arduous.

Agenda Setting

Kingdon (1995) has described agenda setting in public policymaking as a function of the confluence of three "streams" of activities: problems, possible solutions to the problems, and political circumstances. In his conceptualization, when all three flow together in a favorable alignment, a window of opportunity (see Figure 3.1) is created through which a policy issue emerges from the pack and activity shifts to the development of legislation to address the issue. Current policies such as those pertaining to environmental protection, licensure of health professionals and healthcare organizations, funding for AIDS research, or increased funding for women's health exist because these issues emerged previously as sufficiently important that policies to address the issues were developed.

However, the mere existence of problems in these areas was not sufficient to ensure the development of legislation intended to address them. The existence of problems, even serious ones with widespread implications (e.g., high costs and uneven access to needed healthcare services), does not invariably lead to policies that address or solve them. There must also be potential solutions to these problems. The probability of a solution depends on the generation of ideas for solving problems, refinement of those ideas, and, ultimately, selection from among the options. While the menus of alternative solutions to problems vary in size and quality, there are almost always alternative possible solutions to the problems that face policymakers. Without at least one solution, however, issues do not advance in the policymaking process. When there are many alternatives, each with its opponents and proponents, as is often the case, advancement can be slowed as the relative merits of the competing alternatives are considered.

The existence of problems and potential solutions to them are not sufficient to advance issues along in the policymaking process. A political will is also necessary to have this happen. This third variable in creating a window of opportunity for legislation to be developed includes such factors as the public attitudes, concerns, and opinions surrounding an issue; the preferences and relative ability to influence political decisions of various groups that have an interest in the issue; the positions of key political leaders in the executive and legislative branches of government on the issue; and the other competing items on the policy agenda. The array of competing items on the policy agenda is a very important political variable. For example, when the nation is involved in serious threats to its national security or its civil order, during a presidential election season, or when a state is in the midst of a sustained recession, health policy will be treated differently than when policymakers are less preoccupied with other urgent concerns.

Creating a political thrust forceful enough to have policymakers attempt to do something substantive about an issue is often the most problematical variable in having it emerge from the pack of competing issues. This elusive element often keeps the window of opportunity closed, preventing active development of legislation to address the issue.

This circumstance is not particularly surprising, in part because the design of the U.S. government lends itself to political stalemate. Out of fear of potential government abuse of power, the nation's founders created a government more suited to inaction than to action (Morone 1990).

Another important factor in explaining why political circumstances so often prevent progression to policy development lies in the nature of the American electorate. While voters usually do not have the opportunity to vote directly on policies, they do vote on policymakers. Thus, policymakers are interested in what the voters want, even when it is not easy to discern what they want. And often it is very difficult to judge the electorate's position on issues. Their opinions are usually mixed. Polls of potential voters can sometimes help sort this all out, but polls are not always straightforward. The voters' propensity to change their opinions complicates judging what they want.

Yankelovich (1992) points out that the public's thinking on difficult problems that might be addressed through public policies evolves through predictable stages, beginning with awareness of the problem and ending with judgments about its solution. In between, the public explores the problem and alternative solutions with varying degrees of success. What voters believe for any particular issue can vary greatly along this continuum of stages.

Eventually, as the agenda-setting process grinds along, situations can emerge in which the existence of a problem is widely acknowledged, in which possible solutions are identified and refined, and in which favorable political circumstances exist. When this confluence occurs, a window of opportunity opens (albeit usually only briefly) through which an issue moves forward and the development of legislation intended to address the issue is initiated (see Figure 3.1). When this happens, policymakers use a dynamic, highly interactive process through which they seek to convert ideas, hopes, and hypotheses into concrete public policies.

The Development of Legislation

This section contains a simplified and abbreviated outline of the very complex process through which legislation is developed at the federal level.[1] With modifications, which vary from state to state, the legislative process in the states is similar in a general sense to the federal process outlined below. The process consists of a carefully ordered set of steps. The tangible final products of the legislative process are laws or statutes. At the federal level, these are first printed in pamphlet form called *slip*

---

1. For readers who have access to the Internet, another useful description of this process can be found by accessing "How Laws are Made" at http://thomas.loc.gov/.

law. Later, laws are published in the *Statutes at Large* and eventually incorporated into the *United States Code*. The series of steps in this process apply whether legislation is completely new or whether, as is so often the case, it represents the amendment of prior legislation.

Step 1: Drafting and introducing legislative proposals. The legislative process begins with legislative proposals, called *bills*, which can be drafted by any senator or representative, usually with the help of their staffs. Proposed legislation can also be drafted by others, including people in the executive branch, private groups such as healthcare associations or other health interest groups, or even individual citizens. No matter who drafts legislation, however, only members of Congress can officially sponsor proposed legislation, and the legislative sponsors are ultimately responsible for the language in the bills they sponsor.

Step 2: Introduction and referral of proposed legislation. Proposed legislation in the form of a bill is introduced by members of the Senate or House of Representatives who have chosen to sponsor or co-sponsor the bill. On occasion, identical bills are introduced in both the Senate and the House of Representatives for simultaneous consideration. When bills are introduced in either chamber of Congress, they are assigned a sequential number (e.g., HR-1 or S-1, based on the order of introduction) by the presiding officer and are then referred to the appropriate standing committee for further study and consideration. The assignment to an appropriate committee depends upon the content of the bill and the jurisdiction of the committees and of their subcommittees. Sometimes the content makes the bill appropriate for more than one committee; in these cases the bill can be assigned to more than one committee either jointly or, more commonly, sequentially.

Both the Senate and House of Representatives are organized into committees and subcommittees. Ideally, this organization facilitates the division of work and the orderly consideration of proposed legislation. In reality, however, the committee structure itself can sometimes present or exacerbate problems, especially those that involve jurisdictional "turf" issues. Health issues frequently fall into this category. Even in the face of such shortcomings, however, the committee structure is a fundamental feature of the development of legislation.

The majority party in each chamber controls the appointment of committee and subcommittee chairpersons. It also appoints the majority of each committee or subcommittee's members and assigns most of the staff for each committee. The chairpersons of committees and subcommittees exert great power in the legislative process because they determine the order and pace at which legislative proposals are considered by their respective committees or subcommittees. By virtue of expert knowledge, the professional staff serving committees and subcommittees are key participants in the legislative process.

Depending upon whether the chairperson of a committee has assigned a bill to a subcommittee, either the full committee or the subcommittee can hold hearings. Members of the executive branch, representatives of interest groups, and other individuals are permitted to present their views and recommendations on the legislation under consideration at these hearings. After such hearings, committee or subcommittee members will mark up the bill, the procedure of amending the bill by going through the bill line by line and making changes. Sometimes when similar bills, or bills addressing the same issue, have been introduced, they are combined in the marking-up process. In cases in which a subcommittee is involved, the subcommittee completes the marking-up process and reports out the bill to the full committee with jurisdiction. When no subcommittee is involved, or after a full committee reviews the work of the subcommittee, the full committee reports out the bill to the floor of the Senate or House for a vote.

Step 3: House or Senate floor action on proposed legislation. Following approval of a bill by the full committee with jurisdiction, the bill is discharged from the committee along with a bill report that contains a great deal of information about the bill's history and the committee's reasons for its approval. The House or Senate receives the bill from the relevant committee and places it on the legislative calendar for floor action. A bill can be further amended in debate on the floor of the House or the Senate. However, because both chambers place such great reliance on the committee process, amendments to bills proposed from the floor require considerable support.

Bills, once passed in either the House or Senate, are sent to the other chamber, where they repeat the process of being referred to a committee and perhaps then to a subcommittee, which goes through its own process of hearings, mark-up, and eventual action. If the bill is again reported out of committee, it goes to the involved chamber's floor for a final vote. If passed in the second chamber, any differences in the House and Senate versions of a bill must be resolved before the bill is sent to the White House for action by the president. The Congress has a special procedure for ironing out any differences in the versions of bills passed by the House and Senate.

Step 4: Conference committee action on proposed legislation. The procedure for resolving differences in a bill that has been passed by both chambers of the Congress is the establishment of a conference committee that is charged to resolve the differences. Conferees usually are the ranking members of the committees that reported out the bill in each chamber. If they can reach agreement on resolving the differences, a conference report is written and this is then voted on by both houses of the Congress. In the event that the conferees cannot reach agreement, or if either house does not accept the report, the bill dies. If both chambers accept the conference report, the bill is sent to the president for action.

Step 5: Presidential action on proposed legislation. The president has several options regarding proposed legislation that has been approved by both the House and Senate. The bill can be signed, in which case it immediately becomes law. The bill can be vetoed by the president, in which case it must be returned to Congress along with an explanation of the basis for rejection. By two-thirds vote in both houses of the Congress, a presidential veto can be overridden. The president's third option is neither to veto nor to sign the bill. In this case, the bill becomes law in ten days, but the president has made a political statement of disapproval of the legislation. Finally, when proposed legislation is received by the president near the close of a Congress, the president can pocket veto the bill by doing nothing until the Congress is adjourned, in which case the bill dies.

The Policy Implementation Phase

As depicted in Figure 3.1, the formulation phase (making the decisions that lead to legislation) and the implementation phase (taking actions and making additional decisions necessary to implement legislation) of the public policymaking process are bridged by the formal enactment of legislation. Enactment shifts the focus from formulation to implementation. The relationship between policy formulation and policy implementation is simple, direct, and very important. Policies, once enacted as laws, must be effectively implemented if they are to have any chance of exerting their intended effect.

In the implementation phase, much, although not all, of the responsibility in policymaking shifts from the legislative branch of government to the executive branch. Because implementation responsibility rests so heavily within the executive branch, many of its departments, such as the Department of Health and Human Services and the Department of Justice, are involved, as are a number of independent federal agencies such as the Environmental Protection Agency, the Consumer Product Safety Commission, and the FTC. As was noted earlier, these executive branch agencies exist to implement the policies embodied in legislation.

Although the executive branch bears most of the responsibility for implementing policies, the legislative branch maintains an oversight responsibility and often a continuing appropriations responsibility in the implementation phase. Oversight of the executive branch's implementation of policies enacted by the legislative branch is actually mandated in the Legislative Reorganization Act of 1946. Generally, according to the Congressional Research Service (1984), oversight is intended to accomplish the following distinct goals:

- ensure that the implementing organization adheres to congressional intent;
- improve the efficiency, effectiveness, and economy of government's operations;
- evaluate program performance in an ongoing way;
- assess the ability of implementing organizations and individuals to manage and accomplish implementation, including investigation of alleged instances of inadequate management, waste, fraud, dishonesty, or arbitrary action; and
- ensure that the implementation of policies reflects the public interest.

Legislative branch oversight of the executive branch's implementation of policies is accomplished through several means. One powerful technique is through the funding appropriations that Congress must make for the continuing implementation of many policies. Although some health policies, such as the Medicare program, are entitlements, many others require annual funding through appropriations acts. Examples include the research programs of the NIH, the Department of Veterans Affairs' health activities, and the activities of the U.S. Public Health Service, and the FDA. Review by the appropriations committees is an important means of oversight of the implementation performance of these organizations. Other oversight techniques include direct contact between members of Congress and their staffs with executive branch personnel who are involved in implementing policies, hearings on the performance of implementing organizations, and the use of oversight agencies created by Congress to help with this process (Nadel 1995). These agencies include the General Accounting Office, the Congressional Research Service, the Office of Technology Assessment, and the Congressional Budget Office.

There is also a judicial dimension to the implementation phase. Administrative law judges hear the appeals of people or organizations that are dissatisfied with the way implementation of policies affects them. Legislation, as well as the rules made by those responsible for its implementation, can be challenged in the courts.

As was noted above, some of the decisions made within the executive branch organizations, as they implement policies, become policies themselves. For example, rules and regulations promulgated in order to implement a law are policies just as are the laws whose implementation the rules support. Similarly, decisions made in the judicial branch regarding the applicability of laws to specific situations or regarding the appropriateness of the actions of implementing organizations are decisions that are themselves public policies.

Policy implementation involves managing human, financial, and other resources in such ways that the objectives and goals embodied in enacted legislation can be achieved by those responsible for implementation. The most important point in understanding policy implementation, as part of the larger cycle of policymaking, is that it should be viewed primarily as a management process. Depending upon scope and complexity, implementation can be fairly simple and straightforward or can require massive managerial effort. President Lyndon B. Johnson observed that the preparations made for implementing the Medicare law represented "the largest managerial effort the nation (had) undertaken since the Normandy invasion" (Iglehart 1992).

The implementation phase of public policymaking includes two separate, but interrelated, sets of activities: rulemaking and policy operation (see Figure 3.1). Both sets of activities are described below.

Rulemaking

Enacted legislation seldom contains enough explicit language on how the legislation is to be implemented to guide the implementation process completely. Rather, laws are often vague on implementation details, leaving it to the implementing organizations to promulgate the rules needed to guide their implementation. While the means through which the rules and regulations necessary for the implementation of laws are established varies among the levels of government, there are more similarities than differences. The federal process serves as a prototype and is the focus here.

The promulgation of rules, as a formal part of the implementation phase, is itself guided by certain rules. Key among these is the requirement that the organization responsible for implementing a law publish a Notice of Proposed Rule Making (NPRM) in the *Federal Register*. An NPRM is effectively a draft of a rule or set of rules under development. Publication of this notice is an open invitation to all those in a relevant policy community—that is, those with an interest in the rules and regulations applicable to implementing a particular law—to react to proposed (draft) rules before they become final. Changes in proposed rules often result from this procedure. It is one of the most active points of involvement for those who seek to influence the policymaking process. This fact will be considered in detail in Chapter 5.

On occasion, special provisions may be made regarding the development of rules and regulations, especially when their development is anticipated to be unusually difficult, seems prone to spawn severe disagreements and conflicts, or when rules and regulations are anticipated to be subject to continuous revision. For example, after passage of the Health Maintenance Organization Act in 1973, its implementors organized a series of task forces, including on them some members drawn from outside the implementing organization, to help develop the proposed rules for implementing the law. This strategy produced more acceptable rules for those who would be affected by them than might have otherwise been the case.

Another strategy that is used to support rulemaking is the creation of advisory commissions to assist with the effort. For example, following enactment of the 1983 Amendments to the Social Security Act that established the prospective payment system for reimbursing hospitals for the care of Medicare beneficiaries, Congress established the Prospective Payment Assessment Commission (ProPAC) to provide nonbinding advice to the Health Care Financing Administration (HCFA) in implementing the reimbursement system. Later, a second commission, the Physician Payment Review Commission (PPRC), was established to advise Congress and the HCFA on payment for physicians' services under the Medicare program. These commissions are quite useful in helping the HCFA to make required annual decisions about reimbursement rates, fees, and other variables in the operation of the Medicare program.

Policy Operation

After laws are enacted, and after initial rules necessary for implementing them have been promulgated, the implementation phase enters a policy operation stage (see Figure 3.1). Here, implementors typically seek to fulfill the mandates inherent in the laws they are responsible for implementing and to do so by following the rules and regulations promulgated to guide implementation. Of course there is always the possibility that some individuals with implementing responsibilities will disagree with the purposes of enacted laws and will seek to stall, alter, or even subvert the laws in their implementation phases. The power of those with implementation responsibilities to affect the final outcomes and consequences of policies should not be underestimated. It is a power similar to that possessed by those with operational responsibilities in private sector organizations over the achievement of organizational strategies.

Policy operation involves the actual running of programs and activities embedded in enacted legislation. This stage is the domain, although not exclusively, of the appointees and civil servants who staff the government. Two variables are especially important to the successful operation of policies: the policies themselves, and the characteristics and capabilities of the organizations charged with their implementation.

As with any writing that is intended to influence the actions, behaviors, or decisions of others (e.g., legal contracts or procedure manuals), the language and construction of an individual policy play a crucial role in the course and success of its implementation. The effect of the construction of a policy can be felt in both rulemaking and policy operation stages.

Well-constructed policies begin with clearly articulated, meaningful, and achievable goals. Beyond this, they must be based on workable procedural paradigms. Embedded in every policy is a hypothesis: "If a, b, c, and so on are done at time one, then x, y, z, and so on will result at time two" (Thompson 1991, 151). The causal relationship implied in the construction of policies reflects that policies themselves are but means to ends, the ends being the solution of problems. If the hypothesis embedded in a policy is wrong, the policy cannot be effectively implemented because the policy will not solve the problem it is intended to address. It will not matter that its goals are appropriate, or even that they are noble. A third important feature in the construction of policies is the nature and extent of decisions left to the implementing agencies by virtue of explicitly direct language in a statute, by what is not said in a statute, or by confusing or vague language in a statute. While a degree of flexibility in developing the rules and regulations to be used in policy implementation can be advantageous, vague directives included in policies can create problems for those with implementation responsibilities.

Although the way in which a policy is written can have a significant effect on its implementation, so too can the characteristics and capabilities of the implementing organizations. Among the most important are the fit between the implementing organization and the purposes and goals of the policies they are charged to implement; the quality of the implementing organization's leadership; the ability of implementing organizations to work smoothly with other organizations that are involved in implementation; and the appropriateness of the technologies to support their work that are available in the implementing organization (Morone 1992).

No characteristic of an implementing organization is more basic to success than a close fit between the organization and the purposes and goals of the policies it must implement. According to Morone (1992), the keys here include whether the organization is sympathetic to the policy's goals and whether the organization has the necessary resources (i.e., money, personnel, prestige, and skills) to implement the policy effectively.

Especially important among the needed skills are those of the implementing organization's leadership. Necessary support for the implementation task must be garnered and the policy and its implementation must be protected from unwarranted amendments or intrusions by those who do not support the policy. Allies in the legislative branch and among interest groups can be very important to this process, but much of the responsibility rests with the leaders of the implementing organization. They must:

- mold a widely shared internal and external agreement on the implementing organization's purposes and priorities;
- build widespread support for the organization's purposes and priorities among internal and external stakeholders, especially among legislative overseers and relevant interest groups;
- strike a workable balance among the economic and professional interests of the organization's members, its other stakeholders, and the public interest the organization is required to serve; and
- negotiate and maintain effective relationships with other people or organizations who are affected by, or with whom the implementing organization must work closely in carrying out, its policy implementation role.

When more than one organization is involved in the implementation of policies the important issues of interorganizational relationships that have been previously established and the organization's general capabilities to work effectively with other organizations on which they depend to carry out their implementation responsibilities arise. Rarely is a health policy implemented by a single organization or agency, and never when the policy is large in scope. Implementation of the Medicaid program, for example, involves the HCFA working with the Medicaid agencies in each state and with such private sector healthcare organizations as hospitals and nursing homes. The successful implementation of the Medicaid program depends heavily upon the quality of the interactions among these and other organizations.

Implementing organizations rely upon a variety of tools, methods, and technologies to implement policies. Just as policies differ in substantial ways (remember the distinction between allocative and regulatory policies made above), the technologies needed to implement them also differ (Thompson 1991). Regulatory policies require such technologies as those through which implementing organizations prescribe and control certain behaviors of those who are regulated. These technologies include rulemaking, investigatory capacity, and the ability to impose sanctions. Allocative policies require technologies such as those through which implementing organizations deliver income, products, or services. Technologies of this type include properly identifying and targeting recipients or beneficiaries, determining eligibility for benefits, and managing the supply and quality of products and services provided through the policy.

Figure 3.1 shows that the rulemaking and policy operation activities of implementation are related to each other cyclically. This cyclical relationship is quite important. It means that experience gained with the operation of policies can influence the modification of rules and regulations used in the implementation phase. Practically, this means that the rules and regulations promulgated to implement policies can undergo revision (sometimes extensive and continuous) and that new rules can be adopted as experience dictates. This feature of policymaking tends to make the process much more dynamic than it would otherwise be.

The Policy Modification Phase

Policy modification occurs when the outcomes, perceptions, and consequences of existing policies feed back into the agenda-setting and legislation development stages of the formulation phase and into the rulemaking and policy operation stages of the implementation phase to stimulate changes in legislation, rules, or operations. This is shown as the feedback loop in Figure 3.1.

A very important feature of public policymaking in the United States, as it pertains to healthcare, is that most of the public policies that are important to strategymakers in healthcare organizations are the result of modification of prior policies. In fact, so many policies result from the modification of existing policies, and so many of the modifications represent only modest changes, that the entire public policymaking process in the United States has been characterized as a process of incrementalism (Lindblom 1959).

Incrementalism provides a mechanism for compromises to be reached among diverse interests. For some, incrementalism and compromise in policymaking are seen as negatives, implying compromised principles, inappropriate influence peddling, and corrupt deals made behind closed doors. More realistically, however, "in a democracy compromise is not merely unavoidable; it is a source of creative invention, sometimes generating solutions that unexpectedly combine seemingly opposed ideas" (Starr and Zelman 1993, 8).

The major participants in the policymaking process (i.e., policymakers in all three branches of government as well as most organized interest groups) have a preference for incrementalism in public policymaking. This is certainly the case for most members of the health policy community. The primary reason for this preference is that the results and consequences of decisions made incrementally are more predictable and stable than with decisions made less incrementally.

Public policies that pertain to healthcare provide many examples of patterns of incrementally developed policies. For instance, the history of the evolution of the NIH vividly reflects incremental policymaking over a span of more than 50 years. Beginning in the 1930s as a small federal laboratory conducting biomedical research, the NIH has experienced extensive elaboration (the addition of new institutes as biomedical science evolved), growth (its annual budget is now about $12 billion), and shifts in the emphasis of its research agenda (cancer, AIDS, women's health, etc.). Every step in its continuing evolution has been guided by specific changes in policies, each one an incremental modification intended to have the NIH make only marginal adjustments in its actions, decisions, and behaviors.

The policymaking process provides abundant opportunities for the feedback of the outcomes, perceptions, and consequences that result from the implementation of policies to influence the formulation or reformulation of policies. The process also permits the feedback to stimulate the modification of policies in the implementation phase. The results of policy implementation routinely lead to modifications through rulemaking and policy operation activities, often in both concurrently. Such adjustments are directed by the managers of the implementing organizations and are like the activities that managers of all sorts of activities engage in when they seek to control the results of their operations. Standards or objectives are established, operations ensue, results are monitored, and changes are made in operations or objectives, or both when results do not measure up. Such routine operational modifications are inherent in the implementation phase of any policy. They are part of the daily work that occurs within organizations that implement health policies.

In a very real sense the modification phase of the public policymaking process exists because perfection cannot be achieved in the other phases and because policies are established and exist in a dynamic world. Suitable policies are made obsolete by biological, cultural, demographic, ecological, economic, ethical, legal, psychological, social, and technological changes on a routine basis. Modification permits necessary adaptation to such changes and in so doing brings the policymaking process full cycle.

The Utility of the Policymaking Model to Strategymakers in Healthcare Organizations

This chapter began with introduction of the essential notion that strategymakers in a healthcare organization have two very important sets of responsibilities regarding their organization's public policy environment:

- They are responsible for analyzing their organization's public policy environment.
- They are also responsible for influencing this environment.

The model of the public policymaking process presented in this chapter can assist strategymakers in healthcare organizations in fulfilling both sets of responsibilities.

Regarding their analyzing responsibility, the model helps strategymakers understand that it is not enough merely to focus on the product of the process; that is, on policies. They must also develop an understanding of the source of the public policies that affect their organizations. That is, they must understand the larger public policy environment of their organization. The model of the policymaking process depicted in Figure 3.1 can be instrumental in thinking systematically about the public policy environment of a healthcare organization. Chapter 4 focuses on how strategymakers can best approach this challenging responsibility.

Regarding their influencing responsibility, the model of the public policymaking process described in this chapter can be in a very real sense a "map" to the places in the process where influence can be exerted. This use of the model is expanded upon in Chapter 5.

Summary

Public policies are authoritative decisions—made in the legislative, executive, or judicial branches of government—that are intended to direct or influence the actions, behaviors, or decisions of others. When these policies pertain to or influence the pursuit of health they can be thought of as health policies. Public policies can take several forms including laws or specific pieces of legislation, rules and regulations established in order to implement laws or programs, and the judiciary's relevant decisions.

Public policies are made through a highly complex, interactive, and cyclical process that incorporates formulation, implementation, and modification. The process is played out in the context of the political marketplace, where demanders and suppliers of policies interact. The participants in the health policymaking process are diverse, including elected and appointed members of all three branches of government as well as the civil servants who staff the government, and interested individuals and organizations that policies affect. The interests of these participants rarely coincide and are often in conflict, and the activities of any participants always affect and are affected by the activities of other participants. Thus, the public policymaking process is very much a human process, a fact with great significance for its outcomes and consequences.

References

Bice, T. W. 1988. "Health Services Planning and Regulation." In *Introduction to Health Services*, 3rd ed., edited by S. J. Williams and P. R. Torrens, 373–405. New York: John Wiley & Sons.

Brown, L. D. 1991. "Knowledge and Power: Health Services Research as a Political Resource." In *Health Services Research: Key to Health Policy*, edited by E. Ginzberg, 20–45. Cambridge, MA: Harvard University Press.

———. 1992. "Political Evolution of Federal Health Care Regulation." *Health Affairs* 11 (Winter): 17–37.

Coddington, D. C., K. D. Moore, and E. A. Fischer. 1996. *Making Integrated Health Care Work*. Englewood, CO: Center for Research in Ambulatory Health Care Administration.

Feldstein, P. J. 1988. *The Politics of Health Legislation: An Economic Perspective*. Ann Arbor, MI: Health Administration Press.

Iglehart, J. K. 1992. "The American Health Care System: Medicare." *New England Journal of Medicine* 327 (12 November): 1467–72.

Kingdon, J. W. 1995. *Agendas, Alternatives, and Public Policies*, 2nd ed. New York: HarperCollins College Publishing.

Lindblom, C. E. 1959. "The Science of Muddling Through." *Public Administration Review* 14 (Spring): 79–88.

Lumsdon, K. 1992. "HIV-positive Health Care Workers Pose Legal, Safety Challenges for Hospitals." *Hospitals* 66 (20 September): 24–32.

Marmor, T. R., and J. B. Christianson. 1982. *Health Care Policy: A Political Economy Approach*. Beverly Hills, CA: Sage Publications.

Morone, J. A. 1990. *The Democratic Wish: Popular Participation and the Limits of American Government*. New York: BasicBooks.

———. 1992. "Administrative Agencies and the Implementation of National Health Care Reform." In *Implementation Issues and National Health Care Reform*, edited by C. Brecher, 47–72. Proceedings of a conference sponsored by the Robert F. Wagner Graduate School of Public Service, New York University, June 1992.

Nadel, M. 1995. "Congressional Oversight of Health Policy." In *Intensive Care: How Congress Shapes Health Policy*, edited by T. E. Mann and N. J. Ornstein, 127–42. Washington: American Enterprise Institute and The Brookings Institution.

Shortell, S. M., R. R. Gilles, D. A. Anderson, K. A. Erickson, and J. B. Mitchell. 1996. *Remaking Health Care in America: Building Organized Delivery Systems*. San Francisco: Jossey-Bass Publishers.

Starr, P., and W. A. Zelman. 1993. "Bridge to Compromise: Competition Under a Budget." *Health Affairs* 12 (Supplement): 7–23.

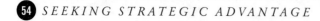

Thompson, F. J. 1991. "The Enduring Challenge of Health Policy Implementation." In *Health Politics and Policy*, 2nd ed., edited by T. J. Litman and L. S. Robins, 148–69. Albany, NY: Delmar Publishers Inc.

U.S. Congressional Budget Office. 1991. *Rising Health Care Costs: Causes, Implications, and Strategies*. Washington, DC: U.S. Government Printing Office.

Williams, S. J., and P. R. Torrens. 1993. "Influencing, Regulating, and Monitoring the Health Care System." In *Introduction to Health Services*, 4th ed., edited by S. J. Williams and P. R. Torrens, 377–96. Albany, NY: Delmar Publishers Inc.

Yankelovich, D. 1992. "How Public Opinion Really Works." *Fortune* (5 October): 102–8.

4

Analyzing Public Policy Environments

As has been discussed, the external environments of healthcare organizations include many variables that can influence their strategymaking and, ultimately, their organizational performance. In addition to public policies, organizations are routinely affected by market forces and the moves of their competitors, as well as by biological, cultural, demographic, ecological, economic, ethical, legal, psychological, social, and technological developments. Although all of these environmental variables should be analyzed by strategymakers, and taken into account in their strategymaking, this chapter concentrates on the task of analyzing public policy environments.

Strategymakers in healthcare organizations should be concerned about their ability both to analyze and influence their public policy environments because the relationships between public policies and these organizations is direct and very important. For example, healthcare organizations routinely see the effect of public policies on their revenues, their licenses to operate, and their markets. The support of the technologies they use (or not) and their relationships to other organizations are also influenced by the effect of public policies.

Perhaps the clearest way to visualize the depth and magnitude of the relationship between a healthcare organization's public policy environment and its organizational performance is to recognize that the ultimate performance outcomes achieved by the organization—whether measured in terms of financial strength, reputation, growth, quality, competitive position, services provided, or other parameters—always begin with and are heavily influenced by the nature of the opportunities and threats provided by or imposed on the organization from its external environment.

Although they represent only one component of the external environments that encircle healthcare organizations, public policies are extremely important components. As Figure 4.1 illustrates, public policies,

Figure 4.1 The Relationship Between an Organization's External
Environment and Its Performance

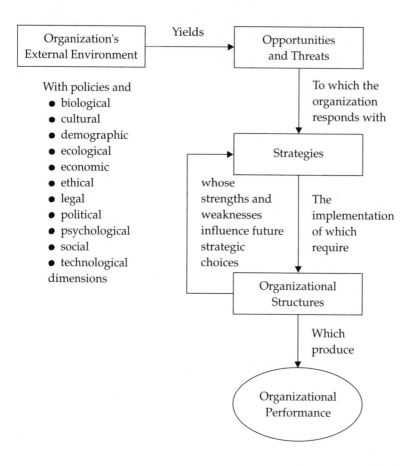

Source: *Health Policymaking in the United States* (p. 135), 1994 by B. B. Longest, Jr. Reprinted by
permission of AUPHA/Health Administration Press.

along with the other variables in an organization's external environment,
provide the organization with a set of opportunities and threats to which
it can—indeed, must—respond.

Organizations respond to the threats and opportunities presented
by their external environments with strategies and with organizational
structures created to carry out the strategies. Strategies and structures
are determinants of organizational performance. But the series of decisions and activities that culminate in organizational performance are
triggered by the opportunities and threats that an organization faces.
And these opportunities and threats are the direct result of conditions in

the organization's external environments, including the public policies that affect it.

Given the importance of organizations' external environments to their ultimate performance, including public policies, strategymakers in most healthcare organizations develop strong operational commitments both to discerning the effects of policies, which they accomplish through effective environmental analysis, and to influencing the policies that affect their organizations. Strategymakers pursue these dual commitments by developing information about policies in advance so that preparations and adjustments can be made, and by seeking to influence the formulation, implementation, and modification of relevant policies. The responsibilities to analyze their public policy environments effectively and what strategic managers can do about fulfilling this responsibility is the focus of this chapter. Chapter 5, in turn, is devoted to the issues involved when strategymakers seek to influence the public policymaking process to their organizations' strategic advantage.

The Importance of Analyzing Public Policy Environments

How much attention should strategymakers in healthcare organizations devote to analyzing their public policy environments? As shown in Chapter 2 (see Figure 2.1), the strategymaking process begins with a situational analysis that includes both external and internal environmental analyses. These analyses are the precursors to the other steps in the strategic management process: strategy formulation, strategic implementation, and strategic control activities. However, it is likely that environmental analyses are not equally important for all strategymakers in healthcare organizations. This is true for overall environmental analyses, and it is true for analyses directed specifically to public policies.

The relative importance of analyzing public policy environments for strategymakers can be gauged by the answers to several questions adapted from A. H. Mesch (1984). The questions are:

- Do public policies influence the organization's capital allocation decisions or its strategic plans for services and markets?
- Have previous strategic plans been scrapped or substantially altered because of changes in public policy?
- Is the organization's industry becoming more competitive? More marketing-oriented? More technology dependent?
- Does the interplay between public policies and the other variables in the organization's external environment seem to be influencing strategic decisions?

- Are the organization's strategic managers displeased with the results of past strategic planning? In particular have there been surprises resulting from changes in public policies that affected the organization?

If the answer to even one of these questions is "yes," then an organization's strategymakers should take their analysis of the public policy environment seriously. If the answer to any three or more of the questions is "yes," then they should consider analysis of their public policy environment to be absolutely imperative and should devote whatever available resources they can to ensuring that the analysis is effectively conducted.

The Potential Benefits of Analyzing Public Policy Environments

Another way of thinking about the importance of analyzing an organization's public policy environment is to focus on the benefits this process might provide to strategymakers in the organization. Such analyses, if they are effectively conducted, can help strategymakers:

- classify and organize complex information about the public policy-making process and about public policies that can or might affect their organization;
- identify and assess current public policies that do or will affect their organization;
- identify and assess the formulation of emerging public policies or amendments to existing policies that might eventually affect their organization;
- speculate in a systematic way about public policies that might emerge in the future and affect their organization; and
- link information about public policies to their organization's strategies and foster strategic thinking within the organization.

These potential benefits to effective strategymaking in healthcare organizations are quite substantial. They may well determine the difference between strategic success or failure, perhaps even between organizational survival and demise in the complex and often hostile environments many contemporary healthcare organizations face.

Limitations in Analyzing Public Policy Environments

Although significant benefits can flow from careful analyses of healthcare organizations' public policy environments, there are certain limitations inherent in these analytical efforts. These should be kept in mind as strategymakers consider the importance of these analyses to their organizations. These limitations include the facts that strategymakers:

- cannot foretell the future through analyses of public policy environments; at best only informed opinions and guesses about the future can be made;
- cannot possibly see every aspect of the policymaking process, or, generally, even be aware of every public policy that will affect their organizations;
- may effectively discern public policies or emergent ones, but be unable to interpret correctly the effect of the policies on their organizations; and
- may effectively discern and interpret the effect of policies, but find their organizations unable to respond appropriately.

A final, and very significant, limitation in the analysis of public policy environments has been identified by Duncan, Ginter, and Swayne (1995), who believe that "perhaps the greatest limiting factor in external environmental analysis is the preconceived beliefs of management. In many cases, what managers already believe about the industry, important competitive factors, or social issues inhibits their ability to perceive or accept signals for change. Because of each manager's beliefs, signals are ignored that do not conform with what he or she believes. Despite long and loud signals for change, in some cases organizations do not change until 'the gun is at their head,' and then it is often too late" (86).

Although there are substantial limitations to what can be expected from analysis of the public policy environments of healthcare organizations, strategymakers in most of them derive enough benefits from doing so to justify their analyzing efforts and to committing substantial resources to the task. Attention is next turned to the question of who is responsible for environmental analyses in healthcare organizations and then to the details of the analytical task itself.

Responsibility for Analyzing Public Policy Environments

Managers who bear strategic responsibilities in healthcare organizations are responsible for the analysis of public policy environments for these organizations, although they typically rely on other people to implement the analyses. It is useful to remember that management work varies in healthcare organizations by the organizational level at which it takes place. Typically, management work is divided into three levels: senior level, middle level, and first level. The work of managers at these different levels varies because their responsibilities differ, as do the resources at their disposal and the combinations of skills they need to perform their work well.

Senior-level managers sit at the top of their organizations and are responsible for the organization's overall performance and condition. Carrying titles such as president, chief executive officer, senior vice president, and in some organizations vice president, senior-level managers occupy, along with their organization's governing boards, what Mintzberg (1983) calls the strategic apex of their organizations. These people set the strategic direction of the organizations they manage. They are responsible for the development of their organizations' objectives and for the organizational strategies that pursue these objectives. Senior-level managers also bear the responsibility for the analysis of public policy environments, as well as the analysis of other components of the external environment as these affect strategic decisions. In short, they must play the strategymaking and strategic management roles in their organizations (Longest 1996).

People who play strategic roles in organizations must think about adapting their organization to its external challenges and opportunities, including relevant public policies. Such adaptation begins with discerning important environmental information. In order to do so, strategymakers identify and follow relevant developments, trends, events, and possible events in their environments that may have strategic consequences for their organizations. But good environmental analysis includes more than merely discerning important information. It also includes organizing and evaluating the information in order to plot the issues that are likely to affect their organizations significantly. To do all of this well usually requires that people in the strategic apex of an organization have the assistance of others. Organizations able to do so typically build into their structures some formal means of accomplishing the environmental analysis functions. However, organizations of all types, including health-care organizations, tend to find rather idiosyncratic solutions to the task of organizing their environmental analysis efforts and activities. Most of them do, however, include in varying ways the specific capability to analyze their external environments in their organization designs.

Building Organizational Capability to Support Public Policy Environment Analysis

Organization designs intended to accommodate the environmental analysis responsibilities that the strategymakers of healthcare organizations have about their public policy environments reflect the well-established history of strategic planning in these organizations (Peters 1985). The management literature is replete with recommendations to create specialized administrative units in organizations, including healthcare organizations, for the purpose of conducting environmental analyses (Ansoff 1980; Porter 1980; Wilson 1982; Lenz and Engledow 1986; Duncan, Ginter, and Swayne 1995). Without exception, these recommendations envision the analyses of public policy environments to be conducted as parts of larger sets of overall environmental analysis responsibilities of such units. Furthermore, these recommendations typically include having the environmental analysis units or activities embedded in departments or units with larger corporate planning, strategic planning, marketing, or public affairs responsibilities.

In important research on this subject, Lenz and Engledow (1986) studied a set of ten organizations to determine how they organized for environmental analysis activities. The organizations chosen for the study were in different industries and were selected for the study specifically because they were considered to be at the "leading edge" of environmental analysis practices. These organizations varied considerably as to where within their designs the environmental analysis activities were housed. There were no apparent contingent relationships between the designs and such factors as the organizations' sizes, their basic strategies, or other aspects of their organization designs.

Healthcare organizations, at least those with the necessary resources, typically build into their structures some formal means of accomplishing the environmental analysis functions, although like organizations in many other industries, they tend to find unique approaches to the task. Commonly, the designs build the activities associated with analyzing public policy environments into the larger workloads of units that are designed to conduct generic environmental analyses, units or departments that also are responsible for overall strategic planning or public affairs. From both efficiency and effectiveness perspectives, this is an appropriate design, in view of the methodological similarities involved in analyzing any part or component of an organization's external environment and because of the close interrelationships between environmental analysis and the conduct of the strategymaking process.

The place where an organization chooses to structure the department will vary depending upon whether it assigns environmental analysis responsibility and authority as a line or staff department. Using Figure 4.2 as a template, a strategic planning department that is organized as a staff department would be attached in an advisory or support capacity to one of the line units. In this case, it might be as a staff department reporting directly to the president or one of the vice presidents shown in the organization chart.

Figure 4.2 A Prototype Healthcare Organization Chart

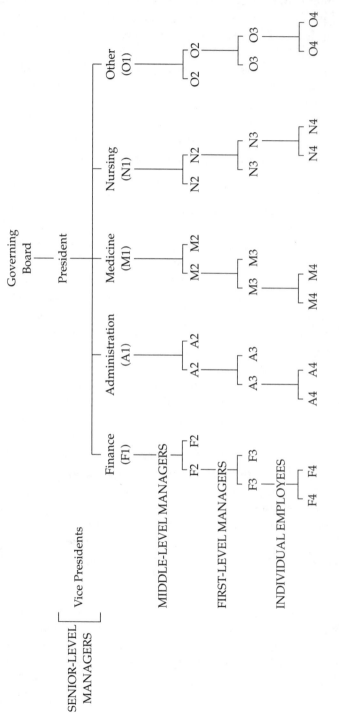

Source: *Health Professionals in Management* (p. 172), 1996 by B. B. Longest, Jr. Reprinted by permission of Appleton & Lange.

A strategic planning department that is organized as a line department or unit could fit on the same line as Finance, Administration, Medicine, and Nursing in the chart in Figure 4.2 and would have its own vice president of strategic planning. Increasingly, healthcare organizations are adopting the line model for these activities (Rakich, Longest, and Darr 1992).

No matter how organizations organize themselves to carry out environmental analyses, the process itself is rather well defined and, as will be seen in the next section, is essentially similar across all types of organizational settings.

The Process of Analyzing Public Policy Environments

It is important to remember that the analyses of public policy environments for healthcare organizations are only parts of larger situational analyses, which are, themselves, parts of still larger strategymaking and strategic management processes in these organizations. It may be useful to go back to Chapter 2 and review Figure 2.1. This review will remind readers that the situational analysis stage of the strategymaking process has two components.

The process includes an external environmental analysis through which strategymakers determine the opportunities and threats facing their organizations as a result of events and variables in their external environments. These events and variables include, but are not limited to, their public policy environments. In fact, the external environments of organizations include all the factors outside their boundaries that can influence their performance. Public policies are certainly among the factors; however, as has been noted in prior chapters, biological, cultural, demographic, ecological, economic, ethical, legal, psychological, social, and technological factors are also relevant and must be routinely analyzed if they are to be taken into account in an organization's strategies.

The strategymaking process examined in Chapter 2 also includes an internal environmental analysis through which strategymakers seek to determine the internal strengths and weaknesses of their organizations and to do so in the contexts of the philosophies, cultures, and objectives of their organizations. The focus of this chapter, however, is restricted to the external environmental analyses, specifically to analyses of the public policy environments of healthcare organizations.

In conducting an analysis of a healthcare organization's public policy environment, its strategymakers can use any of a variety of tools and techniques including trend identification and extrapolation, expert opinion gathered through the Delphi technique or focus groups, and scenario development. No matter which of these techniques is used, it is most productively applied within the framework of a five-step process that is useful in analyzing any organization's external environments, including its public policy environment. Four of the steps in this process are routinely considered in the general strategic management literature (Fahey and Narayanan 1986) and have been adapted for use in healthcare organizations by Duncan, Ginter, and Swayne (1995). A fifth step has been added to their list below.

The interrelated steps in conducting analyses of public policy environments that were briefly described in Chapter 2 are:

- environmental scanning to identify strategic public policy issues (i.e., specific public policies as well as the problems, possible solutions to the problems, and political circumstances that might eventually lead to actual decisions that could affect the organization);
- monitoring strategic public policy issues identified;
- forecasting or projecting future directions of strategic public policy issues;
- assessing implications of the strategic public policy issues for the organization; and
- diffusing results of the analysis of the public policy environment among those in the organization who can help formulate and implement its strategies.

The sequential relationships among these steps are shown in Figure 4.3. Each of the steps is examined in turn in the following sections.

Environmental Scanning to Identify Strategic Public Policy Issues

Environmental scanning activities involve strategymakers acquiring and organizing strategically important information from their organization's external environment. This step properly begins with a careful consideration by strategymakers of what they believe to be strategic public policy issues. It is useful to remember the definition of public policies given earlier: They are authoritative decisions—made in the legislative, executive, or judicial branches of government—that are intended to

Figure 4.3 Steps in Analyzing Public Policy Environments

SCANNING→MONITORING→FORECASTING→ASSESSING→DIFFUSING

direct or influence the actions, behaviors, or decisions of others. When these decisions influence in any way the strategic actions, behaviors, or decisions of healthcare organizations' strategymakers, then they can be thought of as strategic public policies. The set of such strategic public policies—that is, policies that directly or indirectly influence the strategies of healthcare organizations—constitutes a very large set of decisions. Remember that some of these decisions are codified in the statutory language of specific pieces of legislation. Others are the rules and regulations established in order to implement legislation or to operate government and its various programs. Still others are the judicial branch's relevant decisions.

The large set of public policies of strategic importance to healthcare organizations, however, represents only part of what must be considered strategic public policy issues. The problems, potential solutions to the problems, and political circumstances that might align to lead to policies must also be considered important strategic public policy issues. These factors must also be taken into account in complete analyses of public policy environments. Thus, effective scanning of the public policy environment for any healthcare organization involves identifying specific policies (decisions) that are of strategic importance to the organization, and it involves identifying emerging problems, possible solutions to them, and the political circumstances that surround them that could eventually lead to policies. Together, these form the set of strategic public policy issues that should be scanned.

As managers scan their public policy environments, their considerations about what issues are of strategic importance have been described variously as being largely "judgmental," "speculative," or "conjectural" (Klein and Linneman 1984). Obviously, this makes the quality of the judgments, speculations, and conjectures about which of the issues being scanned are of strategic significance quite important. For this reason, it is useful to have more than one person making these judgments. An ad hoc task force or a committee of people from within the organization is one widely used approach to having multiple people render their collective opinions. Another popular approach is to use outside consultants because organizations can benefit from such expert opinions and judgments as to what is strategically important in their environments. It is also possible to use any of several more formal expert-based techniques. The most useful among these are the Delphi technique, the nominal group technique, brainstorming, focus groups, and dialectic inquiry (Duncan, Ginter, and Swayne 1995; Webster, Reif, and Bracker 1989; Delbecq, Van de Ven, and Gustafson 1986; Jain 1984; and Terry 1977). The starting point in any scanning activity, no matter who is scanning or which techniques might be employed, is the question of who and what to scan.

Who and What Should Be Scanned?

Generically, policymakers in federal, state, and local levels of government and those who can influence their decisions—whether through shaping conceptualization of problems and their potential solutions or through impact on the political circumstances that help drive the policymaking process—are the proper focus of scanning activities. The focus can be refined for particular strategymakers by defining the appropriate focus of their environmental scanning to be the strategically important policies and the problems, potential solutions, and political circumstances that might eventually lead to policies that affect their organization.

Another way of identifying who and what should be scanned in a public policy environment is to think of the suppliers of relevant public policies, and those who can influence them, as forming the appropriate focus. Because policies can be made in the executive, legislative, and judicial branches of government, the list of potential suppliers of public policies—the policymakers—is lengthy. Members of each branch of government play roles as suppliers of policies in the political market, although the roles are played in very different ways. Each should receive attention in the scanning activity.

Legislators as suppliers: Legislators are key suppliers of public policies, especially of those in the form of statutes or laws. In the policymaking process, legislators play central roles in supplying policies demanded by their various constituencies. Their important positions in the policymaking process makes them necessary targets of scanning attention. Their motives and behaviors make them very interesting and very challenging subjects for scanning. For example, most legislators constantly calculate the benefits and costs of their policymaking decisions and who will receive those benefits and costs. Then, factoring in the interests they choose to serve, they make their decisions accordingly. In so doing, they create winners and losers, with the policy gains enjoyed by some people coming at the expense of others. While it may be an overgeneralization, it is fair to say that for most legislators, reelection is an abiding factor in their decisions and behaviors and they will seek to maximize their own *net* political gains in such situations. That is, they may find that the best thing for them is to permit the winners their victory, but not by a huge margin so as to cushion the effect on the losers. For example, consideration of a policy to increase healthcare services for an underserved population at the expense of other people could result in any number of outcomes: few services at relatively low cost; more services at higher cost; many services at very high cost. Facing such a decision, policymakers might well opt for the provision of a meaningful level of services, but one far below what could have been provided and at a cost below what would have been required for a higher level of services.

Executives and bureaucrats as suppliers: Members of the executive branches of local, state, and federal levels of government also play important roles as suppliers of public policies. Presidents, governors, and mayors, as well as other high-level executives in their administrations, propose policies in the form of ideas for legislation and encourage legislators to enact their preferred policies. Top executives, as well as executives and managers in charge of departments and agencies of government, make policies in the form of rules and regulations used to implement statutes and programs. In so doing, they become direct suppliers of policies. Elected and appointed executives and managers are joined in the rulemaking role by career bureaucrats who also participate in this process and thus become suppliers of policies in the political marketplace. Elected and politically appointed officials of the executive branch typically have reelection concerns that are similar to those of elected legislators. They also calculate the net political gains available through their decisions and actions regarding various policies. As a result, the motivations and behaviors of elected and politically appointed executive branch officials in the workings of the political marketplace are often quite similar to those of legislators. However, there are some important differences between the motivations and behaviors of elected and appointed members of the executive branch of a government and the elected members of its legislature. The most fundamental of these differences, which is of importance to strategymakers in healthcare organizations, derives from the fact that the executive branch generally bears greater responsibility for the state of the economy than does the legislative branch. Presidents, governors, and mayors, and their top appointees, are held accountable for the condition of the economy in the nation or in the various states and cities more explicitly than Congress or state or local legislatures. This concentration of responsibility in the executive branch for the condition of the economy heavily influences the decision making that takes place there.

Because of the close connection between government's budget and the state of the economy, the budget implications (i.e., deficit-increasing or deficit-reducing implications) of every policy decision will be weighed especially carefully in the executive branch. Not infrequently, positions taken by participants in legislative and executive branches on public policies that are of strategic importance to healthcare organizations will differ because members in the two branches attach different degrees of importance to the budget implications of the decisions they face.

As noted earlier, career bureaucrats in the executive branch also participate in rulemaking, making them direct suppliers of policies. They also collect, analyze, and transmit information about policy options and initiate policy proposals in their areas of expertise. In these ways, they are important participants in the policymaking role of the executive branch. Their motivations and behaviors, however, differ from those of legislators as well as from elected and appointed members of the executive branch.

The behaviors and motivations of career bureaucrats are often quite analogous to those of employees in the private sector. Workers in both the public and private sectors seek to satisfy certain personal needs and desires through their work. This can obviously be categorized as serving their self-interest in both cases. But government employees are no more likely to be totally motivated by self-interests than are private sector workers. Most workers in both sectors are motivated by the same mixture of self-interest and public interest (usually called community interest when the reference is to workers in the private sector) that influence elected and appointed government officials.

Having made this point, it is also fair to note that most career bureaucrats see a constantly changing mix of elected and senior government officials (with an equally dynamic set of policy preferences) come and go, while they remain as the most permanent human feature of government. It should come as no surprise that career bureaucrats develop strong senses of identification with their home departments or agencies or that they develop attitudes of protectiveness toward these homes. This protectiveness is most visible in the relationships between government agencies or departments and those with legislative oversight, including authorization, appropriation, and performance review responsibilities, of those departments. Many career bureaucrats equate the well-being of their agencies, in terms of their size, budgets, and prestige, with the public interest. This is obviously not necessarily the case.

The Judiciary as supplier: The judicial branch of government is also a supplier of public policies. For example, whenever a court interprets an ambiguous statute, establishes judicial procedure, or interprets the U.S. Constitution or a state's constitution, it makes policies. These decisions are not conceptually different from those made when legislators enact laws or members of the executive branch establish rules and regulations for the implementation of the laws. All three sets of activities fit the definition of policies in that they are authoritative decisions made within government for the purpose of influencing or directing the actions, behaviors, and decisions of others.

The heart of the judiciary's ability to supply policies lies in its role in interpreting the law. This power includes the power to declare federal and state laws unconstitutional: that is, to declare laws enacted by the legislative and executive branches to be null and void. The judiciary can also interpret the meaning of laws or statutes, an important role because many laws contain vague language, and members of the judiciary can decide how statutory laws are to be applied to specific situations. And particularly important to their role as suppliers of public policies, the courts can exercise the powers of nullification, interpretation, and application to the rules and regulations established by the government's regulatory agencies.

The courts are involved in numerous and diverse areas of public policy that are of strategic importance to healthcare organizations: termination of treatment, environmental responsibilities, approval of new drugs, mental health law, genetics, antitrust, and so on. It is generally acknowledged that because healthcare is so heavily influenced by laws and regulations that the courts are a major factor in the development and implementation of health-related policies (Christoffel 1991).

It is important to remember that the courts include not only the federal court system, but those of the fifty states and the territories. Each of these systems has developed similarly, but each also has many unique features. Each court system has a constitution to guide it, specific legislation to contend with, and its own history of judicial decisions. Although the federal and state courts play significant roles as suppliers of policies, their behaviors and motivations, as well as their roles, differ significantly from the legislative and executive branches. In their wisdom, the drafters of the nation's constitution created the three branches and ensured, under Article III, the judicial branch's independence, at least largely so, from the other branches. An independent judiciary facilitates that all participants adhere to the rules in the policymaking process. Federal judges are appointed rather than elected, and the appointments are for life. Consequently, federal judges, once they occupy these roles, are not subject to the same self-interest concerns related to reelection that many other policymakers must face. This enhances their ability to act in the public interest, although it does not guarantee that they will.

Those who influence the suppliers of public policies: Clearly, participants in the three branches of government, who directly supply public policies of strategic importance to healthcare organizations, should be scanned. However, the focus of scanning is not limited only to the people and organizational units of government. Any policy domain, whether it is healthcare or another, such as defense, education, or welfare, attracts a diverse set of participants, each of whom has some stake in the policies affecting the domain.

Some of the participants in a domain, who are also known as the stakeholders in that domain, demand policies; other participants supply policies. These stakeholders form a policy community whose members share an interest in a common policy domain. Traditionally, the membership of policy communities has included the legislative committees with jurisdiction in a policy domain (e.g., the Ways and Means Committee in the House of Representatives and the Finance Committee in the Senate), the executive branch agencies responsible for implementing policies in the domain (e.g., the Health Care Financing Administration and the Food and Drug Administration), the courts from time to time as circumstances dictate, *and* the private interest groups in the domain (e.g., the American Hospital Association and the American Medical Association). The first three categories have been identified as suppliers of the policies demanded by the fourth category. Because they seek to influence policymaking, and frequently succeed, those who demand public policies that may be of strategic importance to healthcare organizations also should be scanned. This has become an increasingly difficult task.

The health policy domain during the first half of the twentieth century was dominated by a small number of powerful and concordant private sector members. Furthermore, the private sector members of the policy community, notably the American Medical Association (AMA) and the American Hospital Association (AHA), joined later by the American College of Physicians and the American College of Surgeons, generally held a consistent view as to what the appropriate policies should be in this domain. These private sector members of the health policy community found sympathetic partners in the legislative committees and the implementing agencies for the most part. Their shared view of optimal health policy was that government should protect the interests of healthcare providers and not intervene in the financing or delivery of healthcare (Starr 1982; Wilsford 1991; Peterson 1993). The latter half of the twentieth century, however, has been a different story.

Today, the political market for public policies that are of strategic importance to healthcare organizations is a rough-and-tumble place. The original members of the policy community are still active, but fundamental differences have emerged in their views about health policy. Medicine no longer speaks through the single voice of the AMA. Organizations such as the American College of Physicians and the American Academy of Family Physicians can and sometimes do support different policy choices. The AHA now is joined in policy debates by the diverse preferences of organizations representing the specific interests of teaching hospitals, public hospitals, for-profit hospitals, and other subsets of hospitals.

Not only do the traditional members of the health policy community find themselves split over questions of health policy, the community has been considerably enlarged as new interest groups have formed and joined (Salisbury 1990). Business is the major new member. It too is often split in its views on health-related public policies, primarily along large and small employer lines. Other newer members of the health policy community represent consumer interests. But the interests of consumers are not uniform, nor are the policy preferences of their interest groups.

There is no longer a block of homogeneous interests driving health policy decisions. Instead, the health policy community today "is heterogeneous and loosely structured, creating a network whose broad boundaries are defined by the shared attentiveness of participants to the same issues in the policy domain" (Peterson 1993, 409). There is, however, a large difference between shared attentiveness to issues and agreed-upon positions on the issues. The members of the policy network in the health domain today compete with each other, often fiercely, regarding public policies. After all, while some derive benefits from the status quo, or are threatened by changes in it, others very much want to change the status quo because it either harms them or offers them few, if any, benefits.

The contemporary health network of heterogeneous interests is highly and unprecedentedly fluid and unstable. These characteristics of today's health policy community make it very difficult for the suppliers of health policies to discern what the demanders really want, or which of their diverse demands they should attempt to meet. It also presents significant challenges to strategymakers who seek to scan them effectively. Difficult though it may be, mere scanning is not enough. Strategymakers must also take the next step in the environmental analysis process, monitoring public policy issues.

Monitoring Strategic Public Policy Issues

Effectively scanning the public policy environment for any healthcare organization identifies, and may organize into useful categories when appropriate, specific public policies (decisions) that are of strategic importance to the organization. Really effective scanning also does this as well for the emerging problems, possible solutions to them, and the political circumstances surrounding them that could eventually lead to policies. Monitoring is more than scanning: It is the tracking or following of strategically important public policy issues over time (see Figure 4.3).

Public policy issues are monitored because strategymakers, or their support staffs who are doing the monitoring, believe the issues are of strategic importance. Monitoring them, especially when the issues are not well-structured or are ambiguous as to strategic importance, permits more information to be assembled about issues so that they can be clarified and so that the degree to which they are, or the rate at which they are becoming, strategically important can be determined (Fahey and Narayanan 1986; Thomas and McDaniel 1990).

The monitoring activity has a much narrower focus than the scanning activity (Duncan, Ginter, and Swayne 1995) because the purpose in monitoring is to build a database and information around the set of strategically important public policy issues identified through scanning or verified through earlier monitoring. Fewer, usually far fewer, issues will be monitored than will be scanned.

Monitoring is extremely important because it is often difficult to determine whether environmental issues are strategically important. Under conditions of certainty, strategymakers would fully understand strategic issues and all consequential implications for their decisions and actions. However, uncertainty characterizes much about the strategically important issues that healthcare organizations face. Uncertainty, in most aspects of analyzing organizations' external environments, cannot be removed completely. It can, however, be significantly reduced by the acquisition of more detailed and sustained information through effective monitoring. As with scanning, techniques that feature acquiring multiple perspectives and expert opinions can help strategic managers determine what should be monitored; experts, such as consultants, can also be used in the actual monitoring.

Monitoring the public policy environment will affirm for strategymakers a point that was first raised in Chapter 3. One of the central features of public policymaking in the United States, especially so in regard to the nation's health policies, is that the vast majority of contemporary policies spring from a relatively few earlier policies. Many public policies that are of strategic importance to healthcare organizations result from the modification of prior policies. Policies, such as the Medicare program, have histories. In fact, they are frequently "living" history in that many of them continually, and incrementally, evolve through the amendment process. As these changes are monitored, strategymakers can become intimately familiar with the evolutionary paths of the public policies they monitor. Such knowledge can be very valuable as a background in the next step in the analysis process, forecasting changes.

Forecasting Changes in Strategic Public Policy Issues

Effective scanning and monitoring cannot, in and of themselves, provide strategymakers with all the information they need about strategic public policy issues, or about other important aspects of their external environments. Often, if they are to respond to strategic issues effectively, strategymakers need to forecast future conditions or states. This may give them time to formulate and implement successful strategic responses to the issues.

Scanning and monitoring the public policy environment involves searching this environment for signals, sometimes distant and faint, that may be the forerunners of strategically important issues. Forecasting involves extending the issues and their effects beyond their current states. For some public policy issues (e.g., the effect on patient demand of a change in public policy that redefines the eligibility requirements in the Medicaid program), adequate forecasts can be made by extending past trends or by applying a formula of some kind. In other situations, forecasting must rely upon conjecture, speculation, and judgment, although these can be compiled through such systematic means as Delphi panels or focus groups. Sometimes, even sophisticated simulations can be conducted to forecast the future. However, the results of all of these methods are uncertain. It is especially difficult to include in any of these approaches the fact that few strategically important public policy issues exist in a vacuum. There are almost always many issues at work simultaneously, and no forecasting techniques or models that have been developed to date fully account for this fact.

Trend Extrapolation

The most widely used technique for forecasting changes in public policy issues is trend extrapolation (Klein and Linneman 1984). This technique, when properly used, can be remarkably effective and is relatively simple to use. Trend extrapolation is nothing more than tracking a particular issue, and then using the information to predict future changes. The model of public policymaking that was described in Chapter 3 reflects a process through which public policies rarely come as a bolt out of the blue. Instead, they result from linked trains of activities that can span many years (Molitor 1977), and this feature makes the results of the process more predictable than some might believe.

An instructive example of how the trend extrapolation technique can be used, or misused, by strategymakers can be seen in the pattern of the FDA's mean approval times for new drugs during the 1984 to 1994 period (see Figure 4.4). A strategymaker in a pharmaceutical manufacturing firm in 1991 would very reasonably have anticipated that the approval time for a new drug entered into the review process in that year would be at least 30 months. As shown in Figure 4.4, the process had taken more than 30 months in six of the previous seven years. By trend extrapolation,

Figure 4.4 Mean Approval Times for New Drugs, 1984–94

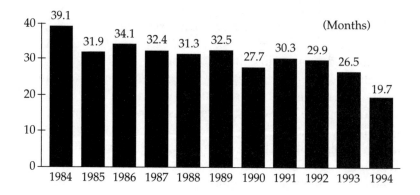

Source: U.S. Food and Drug Administration, 1994.

the 1991 strategymaker would have correctly assumed that a new drug would take at least 30 months to pass through the FDA's review process. The predictability of mean approval times during the 1984 to 1991 period was based on the fact that the FDA's policies during this time were quite stable. With very little changing, the review process took a certain amount of time, and that was that.

For the period beginning in 1992 and beyond, however, the simple trend extrapolation would have led to increasingly incorrect predictions about the mean approval times. The reason for this can be traced to enactment of the Prescription Drug User Fee Act of 1992. This significant new policy requires firms that manufacture or distribute prescription drugs in the United States pay annual user fees to the FDA. The revenues produced by this policy are being used by the FDA to hire more reviewers, streamline the drug review process, and increase its use of information technology. These activities are intended to shorten the time it takes for new drugs to be approved. As can be seen in Figure 4.4, especially in 1994, which was the first full year operating under the new policy, the purpose of the policy is being realized (Barnett 1995).

Trend extrapolation as a technique in environmental analysis must be handled very carefully. It works best under highly stable conditions; under all other conditions it has significant limitations. When used to forecast changes in public policy, it usually permits the prediction of some general trend—such as directional trends in the number of people served by a program or in funding streams—rather than quantification of the trend with great specificity. Significant policy changes, as well as changes in technology, demographics, or other variables, can render the extrapolation of a trend meaningless or misleading. In spite of this, however, predictions about trends through extrapolation can be quite useful to strategymakers in healthcare organizations. For those strategymakers who use it carefully and who factor in the effect of changes such as the introduction of a new or modified policy, trend extrapolation can be a useful technique in forecasting certain aspects of the public policy environments of their organizations.

Scenario Development

Another technique for forecasting the public policy environment is the development, usually in writing, of future scenarios (Leemhuis 1985), which are plausible stories about the future. This technique is appropriate for analyzing environments that include many uncertainties and imponderables. Such features generally characterize the public policy environments of healthcare organizations.

The essence of scenario development is to define several alternative future scenarios, or states of affairs. These can be used as the basis for developing contingent strategies; alternatively, the set of scenarios can be used to select what the strategymakers for an organization consider the most likely future, the one to which they will prepare to respond (Schwartz 1991).

Scenarios of the future can pertain to a single policy issue (e.g., the federal government's policy regarding approval procedures for new medical technology) or to broader-based sets of policy issues (e.g., the federal government's policies regarding healthcare cost containment, medical education and research, or a preventive approach to healthcare). Scenarios can and, in practice, do vary considerably in scope and depth (Venable, Li, Ginter, and Duncan 1994).

As a general rule, when using the scenario development technique in forecasting public policy environments, it is useful to develop several scenarios. Multiple scenarios permit the breadth of future possibilities to be explored. If after the range of possibilities has been reflected in a set of scenarios strategymakers wish to choose one as the most likely scenario, they can do so. But the most common mistake made in using scenario development is to envision too early in the process one particular scenario as "the one true picture of the future" (Fahey and Narayanan 1986).

As an example, consider the scenarios that strategymakers in healthcare organizations might develop for the public policy issue of the federal government's problem of containing overall healthcare costs. It can be assumed that the government will eventually take action to address this problem because of the rate of increase in these costs and their magnitude. Most analysts expect healthcare costs to continue to rise for the foreseeable future. One forecast (Burner, Waldo, and McKusick 1992) has total health expenditures exceeding $1.7 trillion by the year 2000 at which time these expenditures might consume as much as 18 percent of the nation's gross domestic product (GDP), up from its current level of 14 to 15 percent. Already, health spending is greater than for education and defense combined, and as this spending continues to consume a growing share of the nation's resources, fewer resources will be available for other uses. This pattern of extraordinary growth has been and will continue to be an important public policy issue in the environments of healthcare organizations.

A plausible set of scenarios about possible future federal policy initiatives around this issue could include the following, ordered roughly along a dimension of less-to-more radical departure from the status quo:

Scenario 1: Policy incrementalism. In this scenario, federal policies to address the cost problem might include specific, but incremental, actions to reduce the cost of the Medicare and Medicaid programs such as reducing payments to providers, increasing cost-sharing provisions for beneficiaries, and moving beneficiaries into managed care plans. Federal efforts to contain healthcare costs more generally could include such incremental steps as waiving state mandates in health insurance coverage, reducing administrative costs by standardizing insurance claim forms, and instituting reforms to slow the costs of large malpractice awards and the defensive medical practices used to avoid them.

Scenario 2: Managed competition. In this scenario, federal policies could be concentrated on encouraging and facilitating the shift of the healthcare system to a pattern featuring vertically integrated networks of providers competing on the basis of price and quality for large pools of insured people. There may be variations of how this scenario would play out, but its basic components might well have the federal government establishing a standard benefit package and quality standards and perhaps imposing community rating on the establishment of prices.

Scenario 3: Global budgets. In this scenario, federal policies would place caps on total expenditures on healthcare at some predetermined level.

Scenario 4: Single-payer systems. In this scenario, the federal government would assume the role of single payer for all healthcare services, much along the lines of the Canadian approach, and then use its market power to contain costs.

These brief summaries of four scenarios for future federal policy regarding the containment of healthcare costs reflect distinctly different futures. The strategic responses of healthcare organizations to these different futures would also need to be different; responses would need to be specifically tailored to each of the different scenarios. Of course, strategymakers who think they know which scenario will prevail can prepare only for the one they select—and hope they are correct in their forecast. The price of guessing incorrectly, however, can be very high indeed.

Assessing the Strategic Importance of Public Policy Issues

Scanning and monitoring public policy issues, and forecasting future changes in them, are each important elements in a good environmental analysis. However, strategymakers must also concern themselves about the specific and relative strategic importance of the issues they are analyzing. That is, they must be concerned with an assessment or interpretation of the strategic importance and implications of public policy issues for their organizations. Frequently, this involves characterizing issues as threats or opportunities for organizations (see Figure 4.1). Such assessments, however, are far from an exact science. Regarding assessments of the strategic importance of public policy issues, or for other aspects of a healthcare organization's external environment, it has been said that "sound human judgment and creativity may be the bottom-line techniques for a process without much structure" (Duncan, Ginter, and Swayne 1995, 99). Even so, there are several bases upon which the strategic importance of public policy issues can be considered.

Experience with similar issues in the past is frequently a useful basis for assessing a public policy issue's strategic importance. The experience may come from past experiences in the particular organization where an assessment is being made or from other locations that have experienced similar public policy issues. Great variety exists among the states regarding their public policies that affect healthcare and, similarly, the experiences in other countries with various public policies affecting healthcare can be instructive. Other bases for assessments include intuition or best guesses about what particular public policy issues might mean to an organization as well as advice from others who are well-informed and experienced. When possible, quantification, modeling, and simulation of the potential effects of public policy issues being assessed can be useful.

Making the appropriate determination is rarely a simple task, even when all the bases suggested above are considered. Aside from the difficulties encountered in collecting and properly analyzing enough information to fully inform the assessment, personal prejudices and biases can influence those conducting the environmental assessment. Such influences can force assessments that fit some preconceived notions about what is strategically important rather than reflecting the realities of a particular situation (Thomas and McDaniel 1990).

Diffusing the Results of Environmental Analysis into Strategymaking

The final step in the process of analyzing public policy environments in healthcare organizations involves diffusing or spreading the results to all managers who have strategic responsibilities in the organizations so that their strategymaking can be influenced. This step is frequently undervalued as part of the process and, in extreme cases, even overlooked. Unless it is effectively carried out, however, it really does not matter how well the other steps in the process are performed.

As was seen in the model of the strategymaking and strategic management processes that was presented in Chapter 2 (see Figure 2.1), the results of situational analyses, which include both internal and external environmental analyses, feed directly into strategy formulation. Strategymakers are in better positions to formulate their strategies when they are guided by the results of careful environmental analyses conducted for their organizations. Thus, attention must be given to the task of diffusing the results of analyses of public policy environments, as well as many other environments, into the formulation of strategy if the analytical process is to have its desired effect.

There are three basic ways that those who have produced information about the public policy environment of their organization can diffuse this information into the organization's strategymaking process. They can:

- rely upon the power of senior-level managers to dictate diffusion and use of the information, including using coercion or sanctions to see that the information is diffused, and even used, in all the appropriate places in the organization;
- use reason to persuade all those who are involved in strategymaking to use the information; or
- use education of all strategymakers as to the importance and usefulness of their information as a way of improving the chances that the information will influence strategic thinking.

Another way for those who have produced strategically important information about an organization's public policy environment to approach the task of facilitating its diffusion in the organization is to consider top-down edicts versus participative ways of diffusing and encouraging the use of their information. In top-down approaches, which rely upon the use of power, senior-level managers simply announce or dictate that the information is to be used in strategymaking in the healthcare organization. Other participants in the organization are expected to carry out the dictates by including the information in their strategic thinking.

These approaches to diffusing strategically important information have their appropriate uses. For example, a surprise change in a state's reimbursement policy for its Medicaid program might require an immediate strategic shift in healthcare organizations located in that state, leaving little time for anything but a top-down edict to ensure the use of this information in strategymaking. A top-down approach has the advantage of speed, although a major drawback is its disruptiveness and the disenfranchised sense that it gives to those who are making strategic decisions that they are separated from any participation in the production of environmental information upon which to base their decisions.

In participative approaches the use of public policy information is facilitated by having those who must use the information actually participate in its production. Participation can be achieved through such devices as membership on task forces or teams charged to scan, monitor, forecast, and assess the public policy environment. For example, an academic medical center that is concerned about the effect of changes in public funding for medical education might find the necessary strategic adjustments much easier to make if key strategymakers have participated in the production of the information in this area that eventually drives painful strategic decisions about cutbacks in graduate medical education activities.

Diffusion of strategically important information about public policy issues among the strategymakers of organizations brings the model of the analysis process shown in Figure 4.3 to completion. The appropriateness of the fit of any healthcare organization within its external environment depends very heavily on the quality with which this process is conducted.

In fact, given the vital link between healthcare organizations today and the public policies—at all three levels of government—that affect them, no healthcare organization can succeed without a reasonably effective process through which its strategymakers discern and ultimately respond to strategically important public policy issues. But this is only half the task facing the strategymakers regarding their public policy environments. They are also responsible for influencing these environments to the strategic advantage of their organizations. This complex and interesting process is explored in Chapter 5.

Summary

The models of public policymaking and strategic management that were presented in Chapters 2 and 3 have been integrated in this chapter to show

how the results—outcomes, perceptions about the outcomes, and their consequences—of the public policymaking process affect strategymaking in healthcare organizations and, eventually, upon their organizational performance (see Figure 4.1).

Strategymakers in healthcare organizations share—to varying degrees depending upon the impact on them and their organizations—two related areas of concern about their public policy environments. They are concerned about how policies will affect their organizations, giving rise to the need for them to analyze their public policy environments effectively. They also want to have some ability to influence the policies that affect their organizations. This chapter is devoted to the first of these two sets of concerns, that of analyzing public policy environments.

A model of the standard process through which formal analyses of public policy environments, usually as a part of a more general environmental analysis process, are routinely conducted is presented here and forms the organizational framework for much of this chapter (see Figure 4.3). The environmental analysis model includes five interconnected steps: (1) environmental scanning to identify public policy issues of strategic importance; (2) monitoring the strategic public policy issues identified; (3) forecasting or projecting the future directions of strategic public policy issues; (4) assessing the implications of the strategic issues; and (5) diffusing the information produced about public policy issues to strategymakers throughout the organization. Each of the steps in environmental analysis is discussed in turn, and emphasis is given to appropriate techniques that can be used by those responsible to carry out each step effectively.

This chapter emphasizes the fact that in view of the direct connection between the external environments, including public policies, of healthcare organizations and the ultimate performance of these organizations, strategymakers can be expected to develop strong operational commitments both to discerning the effects of policies, as well as to influencing them. In fulfilling their analysis responsibilities, strategymakers seek to develop information about public policies and policy issues in advance of their impact so that strategic adjustments can be made to them. In the next chapter, attention is turned to the second major responsibility strategymakers in healthcare organizations have regarding their public policy environments: how strategymakers can influence the formulation, implementation, and modification of relevant public policies.

References

Ansoff, H. I. 1980. "Strategic Issue Management." *Strategic Management Journal* 1 (2): 131–48.

Barnett, A. A. 1995. "The State of Health Care In America 1995: Pharmaceutical Manufacturers." *Business & Health* 13 (3): 41–46.

Burner, S. T., D. R. Waldo, and D. R. McKusick. 1992. "National Health Expenditures Projections Through 2030." *Health Care Financing Review* 14 (1): 1–29.

Christoffel, T. 1991. "The Role of Law in Health Policy." In *Health Politics and Policy*, 2nd ed., edited by T. J. Litman and L. S. Robins, 135–47. Albany, NY: Delmar Publishers, Inc.

Delbecq, A. L., A. H. Van de Ven, and D. H. Gustafson. 1986. *Group Techniques for Program Planning: A Guide to Nominal Group and Delphi Processes.* Mt. Horeb, WI: Green Briar Press.

Duncan, W. J., P. M. Ginter, and L. E. Swayne. 1995. *Strategic Management of Health Care Organizations*, 2nd ed. Cambridge, MA: Blackwell Publishers.

Fahey, L., and V. K. Narayanan. 1986. *Macroenvironmental Analysis for Strategic Management.* St. Paul, MN: West Publishing Company.

Jain, S. C. 1984. "Environmental Scanning in U.S. Corporations." *Long Range Planning* 17 (2): 117–28.

Klein, H. E., and R. E. Linneman. 1984. "Environmental Assessment: An International Study of Corporate Practices." *Journal of Business Strategy* 5 (Summer): 66–75.

Leemhuis, J. P. 1985. "Using Scenarios to Develop Strategies." *Long Range Planning* 18 (2): 30–37.

Lenz, R. T., and J. L. Engledow. 1986. "Environmental Analysis Units and Strategic Decision-Making: A Field Study of Selected 'Leading Edge' Corporations." *Strategic Management Journal* 7 (1): 69–89.

Longest, B. B., Jr. 1996. *Health Professionals in Management.* Stamford, CT: Appleton & Lange.

Mesch, A. H. 1984. "Developing an Effective Environmental Assessment Function." *Managerial Planning* 32 (1): 17–22.

Mintzberg, H. 1983. *Structure in Fives: Designing Effective Organizations.* Englewood Cliffs, NJ: Prentice-Hall.

Molitor, G. T. T. 1977. "How to Anticipate Public Policy Changes." *Society for the Advancement of Management: Advanced Management Journal* 42 (Summer): 4–13.

Peters, J. P. 1985. *A Strategic Planning Process for Hospitals.* Chicago: American Hospital Publishing.

Peterson, M. A. 1993. "Political Influence in the 1990s: From Iron Triangles to Policy Networks." *Journal of Health Politics, Policy and Law* 18 (2): 395–438.

Porter, M. E. 1980. *Competitive Strategy.* New York: The Free Press.

Rakich, J. S., B. B. Longest, Jr., and K. Darr. 1992. *Managing Health Services Organizations*, 3rd ed. Baltimore, MD: Health Professions Press.

Salisbury, R. H. 1990. "The Paradox of Interest Groups in Washington—More Groups, Less Clout." In *The New American Political System*, edited by A. King. Washington, DC: The American Enterprise Institute.

Schwartz, P. 1991. *The Art of the Long View.* New York: Doubleday/Currency.

Starr, P. 1982. *The Social Transformation of American Medicine.* New York: Basic Books.

Terry, P. T. 1977. "Mechanisms for Environmental Scanning." *Long Range Planning* 10 (3): 2–9.

Thomas, J. B., and R. R. McDaniel, Jr. 1990. "Interpreting Strategic Issues: Effects of Strategy and the Information-Processing Structure of Top Management Teams." *Academy of Management Journal* 33 (2): 288–98.

Venable, J. M., Q. Li, P. M. Ginter, and W. J. Duncan. 1994. "The Use of Scenario Analysis in Local Public Health Departments: Alternative Futures of Strategic Planning." *Public Health Reports* 108 (6): 701–10.

Webster, J. L., W. E. Reif, and J. S. Bracker. 1989. "The Manager's Guide to Strategic Planning Tools and Techniques." *Planning Review* 17 (6): 4–13.

Wilsford, D. 1991. *Doctors and the State: The Politics of Health in France and the United States*. Durham, NC: Duke University Press.

Wilson, I. 1982. "Environmental Analysis." In *Business Strategy Handbook*, edited by K. Albert. New York: McGraw-Hill.

5

Influencing Public Policy Environments

A
s was discussed in previous chapters, public policies are important elements in the environments of all types of organizations, including those involved in healthcare (Buchholz 1989, 1993; Longest; 1988, 1994). One need look no further than the effect of federal Medicare and the combination of federal and state Medicaid policies to see the direct relationship of public policies to healthcare organizations. Beyond this rather obvious example of the effect of public financing policy, there are numerous other public policies that are important elements in the environments of healthcare organizations—policies that fund programs, regulate market-related decisions and behaviors, facilitate medical research and education, and so on.

Thus, as was also noted in the previous chapter, strategymakers in healthcare organizations must be concerned both about effectively analyzing and about influencing their public policy environments. They must seek information about public policies and they must help shape public policies when the policies and their related issues are of strategic importance to their organizations. Typically, such strategymakers seek to ensure that their organizations develop information about relevant policy issues before impact is felt so that strategically sound preparations and adjustments can be made. They do this by using the environmental analysis process and supporting techniques described in the previous chapter.

In addition, they seek to influence the formulation, implementation, and modification of relevant public policies using the techniques described in this chapter. Strategymakers are fulfilling their obligations to manage the relationship between public policy and their organizations only when both their analysis and influence responsibilities are properly met.

The purpose of this chapter is to consider the processes through which strategymakers in healthcare organizations can legitimately and ethically influence the public policymaking process and through this the public policies that are relevant to their organizations. As a means of organizing the discussion about this complex topic, the model of the public policymaking process that was described in Chapter 3 (see Figure 3.1) will be used as a "map" to highlight the places in the process where influence can be exerted.

This chapter also includes a discussion of specific methods to influence the policymaking process at the various points of possible intervention, and it concludes with consideration of the ethical issues inherent in intervening in the public policymaking process. Inclusion of these ethical considerations is important because, although there is nothing innately wrong with exerting influence on the public policymaking process, it must be noted that the process can be tainted by overzealous attempts to influence policies for self-serving purposes.

Before discussing where and how influence can be exerted, some background information on the issue of who is responsible for this activity in healthcare organizations and on the concept of influence in general is presented.

Responsibility for Influencing Public Policy Environments

The authority and responsibility for influencing the public policy environments of healthcare organizations are reserved predominantly for their strategymakers; that is, for their senior-level managers and members of their governing boards. Unlike the analysis of public policy environments as discussed in the previous chapter, influencing public policy environments is typically not assigned to separate departments or units at all, although there may be board committees with oversight responsibilities. Importantly, in most healthcare organizations this stands in contrast to the widespread organization design practice of establishing a department or unit to house the environmental analysis work, along with other strategymaking or strategic planning activities.

Some healthcare organizations do, however, run against the general trend of not assigning responsibility for influencing public policy environments to particular departments. Many of the larger, more complex healthcare organizations, such as academic medical centers or large integrated healthcare systems and networks, establish departments or units specifically charged to conduct work related to influencing the public policy environments of these organizations. These departments are typically called public affairs departments or government affairs or relations departments. Some very large organizations even divide government relations into separate departments, one for the federal government and another for the state government.

When departments that are devoted to influencing public policy environments exist as separate units in an organization's design, they are very likely to be staff units with their own director, who reports to the organization's president or another senior-level manager or strategymaker. Importantly, even when an organization has a staff department that is devoted to influencing its public policy environment, the role of the organization's strategymakers in this process is still vital. Such departments mainly serve to enhance the ability of the organization's strategymakers to succeed in *their* efforts to influence the public policy environment to the organization's advantage.

When actual healthcare organization designs include assigning the analysis and influence duties to different departments or units, it becomes very important that attention be devoted to coordinating both sets of work. The most important way to ensure effective coordination is for strategymakers to insist that the coordination occur. By taking ultimate responsibility, exerting authority over both departments and involving themselves in both sets of work, they can be certain that the expertise and insight held by the people involved in each set of work informs and supports those involved in the other work. For example, valuable information about what aspects of a public policy environment to scan and monitor might well come from people who are intimately involved in trying to influence an organization's public policy environment. Similarly, effective scanning, monitoring, forecasting, and assessing of public policy environments can help establish the most appropriate and promising targets for efforts to influence public policy environments to strategic advantage.

Looking Outside the Organization for Help

The challenges involved for strategymakers to analyze and correctly interpret the effect of relevant issues in their public policy environment and to influence this environment to the strategic advantage of their organization are quite substantial. In large measure, this is the case because so many others are simultaneously seeking to exert their own influence in pursuit of their own preferences in this environment. Strategymakers in healthcare organizations, even very large ones, cannot hope to meet these challenges successfully by relying exclusively on the use of their own internal resources.

Given the extensive and dynamic set of forces and actors at work in their organization's public policy environment, strategymakers must frequently turn for assistance to outside resources in fulfilling both their analysis and influence responsibilities. The primary source of such assistance is the interest groups to which strategymakers and their organizations belong. This aspect of the efforts of strategymakers to succeed at analyzing and influencing the public policy environments of their organizations is so important and so complex that it is treated separately and at length in Chapter 6. In this chapter, the focus is on the mechanisms and techniques available to strategymakers themselves to influence their organization's public policy environment.

No matter how a healthcare organization is designed internally to influence its public policy environment, or how its strategymakers use the help of outside interest groups, the bottom line of exerting influence in public policy environments is that eventually influence must actually be exerted. In the next section, the concept of influence is defined and examined.

The Concept of Influence

Within the context of the political marketplace where public policy-making occurs, as was noted in Chapter 3, many participants seek to further their objectives. Their objectives can be self-interest objectives involving some economic or political advantage or public-interest objectives involving certain participants' perception of what is best for the nation or society. In both cases, the outcome depends greatly on the relative abilities of participants in the exchanges within the marketplace to influence or shape the actions, behaviors, and decisions of other participants. The relevant participants in the public policy environments of healthcare organizations are the "demanders" of public policies (i.e., the strategymakers in the healthcare organizations as well as people inside and outside their organizations who support their efforts) and the "suppliers" of public policies (i.e., those in the legislative, executive, and judicial branches of government with policymaking duties and roles as well as people inside and outside government who exert influence on their decisions).

The exertion of influence in these public policy environments is "simply the process by which people successfully persuade others to follow their advice, suggestion, or order" (Keys and Case 1990, 38). But to have influence one must first have power. Power, whether it occurs in economic or political markets, is necessary because in the context of market relationships and exchanges it is the potential to exert influence. More power means more potential to influence others. Therefore, to understand influence, one must first understand power. Those who wish to exert influence in the political marketplace must first acquire power. But how do they do so, and what are the various sources of power available to them?

Sources of Power in Political Markets

Strategymakers in a healthcare organization, just as those in other types of organizations, have three bases of power that permit them to influence their organization's public policy environment: positional power, the power to reward or coerce others, and the power that derives from the possession of expertise or information. Briefly:

- **Positional power** derives from a person's position in a social system or in an organization; this form of power is also called *formal power* or *authority*. It exists because societies find it advantageous to assign certain powers to individuals to enable them to perform their jobs or fulfill their roles effectively. Thus, elected officials, appointed executives, and judges, as well as strategymakers in healthcare organizations, association professionals, corporation executives, union leaders, individual voters, and many other participants in the political marketplace, possess certain legitimate power that accompanies their social or organizational positions.

- **Power to reward or coerce** others is based on a person's ability to reward compliance, or to punish noncompliance, with the preferred decisions, actions, and behaviors that are sought from others. This form of power stems in part from the positional power that a person holds. Superiors in organizations have this base of power over their subordinates and leaders in Congress have it over the members. Such power stems from the ability to supply or withhold from any person something of value to that person, whether money, vacations, promises of future employment for the person or their family members, and so on.

- **Expert power** derives from possessing expertise or information that is valued by others. Within the political marketplace, such expertise as that necessary for solving problems or performing crucial tasks can be extremely important.

Importantly, for the effective use and effect of power, these three bases in the political marketplace are interdependent, and they can and do complement each other. People whose positions in society or in organizations permit them to use reward power, and who do so wisely, can strengthen their positional power. Similarly, people in positions of power typically have more opportunities to reward or coerce others. Expertise, especially that based on exclusive access to information, is frequently a function of a person's position or access to people in certain positions. Such access can be facilitated through the power to reward or coerce.

Effective participants in the marketplace for policies are those who succeed at translating their power into influence and they tend to be aware of the sources of their power and to act accordingly. Effective participants seem to be those who "understand—at least intuitively—the costs, risks, and benefits of using each kind of power and are able to recognize which to draw on in different situations and with different people" (Morlock, Nathanson, and Alexander 1988, 268).

What enables certain people to use effectively the power to which they have access—that is, to translate power into influence in the political marketplace—is their interpersonal and political skills. It is not enough to have access to power; one must also know how to use it in order to influence others. Mintzberg, perhaps as much as anyone, has recognized this important fact. He attributes success in using power largely to a person's relative political skills, which he defines as:

> the ability to use the bases of power effectively—to convince those to whom one has access, to use one's resources, information, and technical skills to their fullest in bargaining, to exercise formal power with a sensitivity to the feelings of others, to know where to concentrate one's energies, to sense what is possible, to organize the necessary alliances. (Mintzberg 1983, 26)

The Appropriate Focus of Influence

Strategymakers in healthcare organizations should be guided in their efforts to influence policies by focusing on the same activities that they were advised in the previous chapter to use as the focus for their environmental scanning activities. That is, their influencing activities should be guided by the identification of policies that are of strategic importance to their organizations as well as by identification of problems, potential solutions, and political circumstances that might eventually lead to such policies. By focusing in this way, they will seek to influence relevant policymakers strategically in all three branches and in federal, state, and local levels of government. Furthermore, they will extend their efforts to influence to those who have influence with these policymakers. If they are to influence the policymaking process effectively, in addition to influencing policymakers directly, strategymakers must also concern themselves with shaping the conceptualizations of problems, the development of potential solutions to the problems, as well as with the political circumstances that help drive the policymaking process. The suppliers of public policies, and those who can influence them, form the appropriate focus for strategymakers who seek to influence the public policies that will affect their organizations.

In short, strategymakers should exert their influence throughout the entire public policy environment of their organization. A good map to this complex terrain can be very useful.

A Map to Places Where the Public Policymaking Process Can Be Influenced

The model of the policymaking process shown in Figure 5.1, which is a replication of Figure 3.1, can be used to identify the places in the process where strategymakers, either working independently, or, as is more often the case, working in concert with others with similar interests through associations or other collaboratives, can exert influence.

Recall from the earlier discussion in Chapter 3 of the public policymaking process depicted in Figure 5.1 that it includes three interconnected phases:

- policy formulation, which incorporates activities associated with agenda setting and subsequently with the development of legislation;
- policy implementation, which incorporates activities associated with rulemaking and policy operation; and
- policy modification, which exists because perfection cannot be achieved in the other phases and because policies are established and exist in a dynamic world where events and circumstances routinely render existing policies inadequate.

Thinking of Figure 5.1 as a map enables strategymakers to see that the places where efforts to influence public policymaking can be focused are agenda setting, legislation development, rulemaking, and policy operation.

The circular flow of the relationships among the various components of the policymaking process reflects the fact that policymaking is an ongoing process in which almost all decisions are subject to subsequent modification. This feature greatly increases opportunities for strategymakers in healthcare organizations, as well as for others, to influence policies. In effect, those who would influence public policies usually have more than one opportunity to do so.

Techniques for Influencing Public Policymaking

In this section, following the map of places where policies can be influenced shown in Figure 5.1, a variety of techniques through which

Figure 5.1 A Model of the Public Policymaking Process in the United States

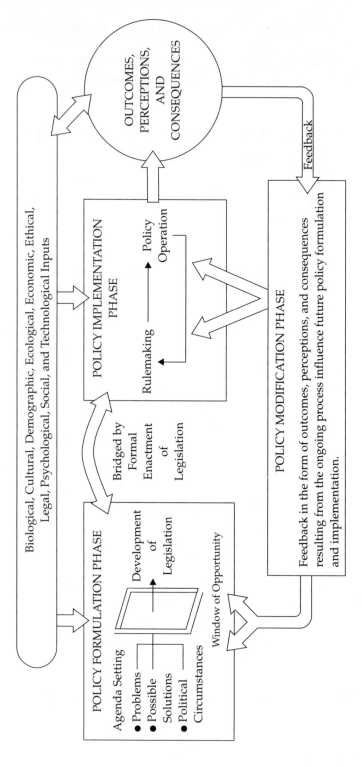

Source: *Health Policymaking in the United States* (p. 160), 1994 by B. B. Longest, Jr. Adapted by permission of AUPHA/Health Administration Press.

strategymakers can exert their influence are identified and described. As will be seen, the techniques differ according to the place in the overall policymaking process where they are used.

Exerting Influence on Agenda Setting

A logical place to begin is on the left side of the policymaking model, where the health policy agenda is shaped by the interaction of problems, possible solutions to the problems, and political circumstances (Kingdon 1995). Strategymakers can exert influence on policymaking by helping to define the problems that eventually become the focus of public policymaking, by participating in the design of possible solutions to these problems, and by helping to create the political circumstances necessary to convert potential solutions into actual policies. In short, policies can be influenced by influencing the factors that establish the policy agenda itself. Each of these important opportunities for influencing policies is considered in turn.

Problems

The scope of problems that can be addressed through the public policymaking process is massive. Even the fraction of all these problems that are of strategic importance to strategymakers in healthcare organizations is large and diverse. After all, health is determined in human populations by several factors acting in combination: the physical, sociocultural, and economic environments in which people live; their lifestyles, behaviors, and genetics; as well as by the type, quality, and timing of healthcare services that they receive (Evans and Stoddart 1994). Problems, real or perceived, in all these areas are of interest to strategymakers. But how do they influence agenda setting around the array of problems in which they have strategic interest? The answer requires a consideration of how the problems that eventually stimulate policymaking come to occupy places on the agenda.

Some problems that drive policymaking emerge because a condition or situation reaches a critical mass or a highly visible or unacceptably troublesome level. Examples include the prevalence of HIV in the population and the growing number of those without health insurance. Another example is the increasing cost to the federal government of the Medicare program and to the states for operating their Medicaid programs. Other problems emerge by virtue of specific events that force attention to them, such as medical waste products washing up on beaches or the discovery of a new drug for treating a relatively rare disorder that is so expensive few people can purchase it on their own. Still other problems are spotlighted by their widespread applicability to many people (e.g., the high cost of prescription medications) or by their sharply focused effect on a small but powerful group (e.g., the high cost of medical education).

Strategymakers in healthcare organizations, because of their positions and of the environmental scanning activities they engage in (as described in Chapter 4), can be among the first to observe certain types of problems, sometimes in their early stages. This gives them an important means through which to help shape the policy agenda. Strategymakers are often well-positioned, especially when they act in concert, to document problems—to gather, catalog, and correlate facts that depict the actual state of a problem and to share this information with policymakers. Problem definition and documentation can exert a powerful influence on the agenda setting that precedes all public policymaking.

An example of problem definition by strategymakers in healthcare organizations that eventually led to a specific policy to address the problem can be seen in the background of Maine's Hospital Cooperation Act of 1992 (Cerne 1993; Kania 1993). Prior to establishment of this legislation, if hospitals in Maine sought to form coalitions to purchase and share expensive technologies or to cooperate in other cost-reducing efforts, they risked violating antitrust laws. As the costs of new technologies grew and as the pressures to contain healthcare costs increased, some of Maine's hospital strategymakers sought legislation that would offer them at least limited protection from the antitrust restrictions so that they could establish cooperative agreements to share expensive technologies or scarce professional personnel to contain healthcare costs.

Through the coordinating efforts of the Maine Hospital Association, the strategymakers' account of the problems they faced in containing costs and of the limitations imposed on cooperative and collaborative solutions by the threat of antitrust sanctions was sufficiently documented. The documentation allowed them to prove the problem and as a result it became part of the public policy agenda in Maine. Eventually, the legislature enacted P.L. 814, the Hospital Cooperation Act of 1992, in response (Michaud 1992).

This policy permitted, under specified circumstances, cooperative agreements among or between hospitals in Maine. In the language of the legislation, "cooperative agreement means an agreement among two or more hospitals for the sharing, allocation or referral of patients, personnel, instructional programs, support services and facilities or medical, diagnostic or laboratory facilities or procedures or other services traditionally offered by hospitals." This policy was enacted through a string of policymaking activities that began with the strategymakers in Maine hospitals documenting to the state legislature that a problem existed that could be at least partially addressed through a policy change.

Possible Solutions

The mere existence of problems, however, no matter how serious or widely acknowledged they are, or how well documented, is not sufficient to trigger the active development of policies to address them. For this to happen, there must also exist possible (or what at least appears to be) solutions to the problems. Enactment of Maine's Hospital Cooperation Act was facilitated not only by the documentation of a problem, but also by the availability of a feasible solution to the problem.

Possible solutions to problems are generated through the development of ideas for solving problems, refinement of the ideas, and, ultimately, selection from among the options. Here again, healthcare strategymakers can be influential in setting the policy agenda as was done in Maine.

Strategymakers in healthcare organizations are, in fact, frequently well positioned to play important analytical and prescriptive roles in determining viable solutions to many problems. Sometimes their organizations can even serve as laboratories for demonstrating the utility of a potential policy solution to a problem. Examples of this abound. The experience of Maine hospitals with their Hospital Cooperation Act has been instructive for healthcare organizations and legislatures in other states regarding this approach as a potential solution to their own similar problems. A rather comprehensive list of healthcare organization-based demonstrations with policy relevance can be found in Shortell and Reinhardt (1992), including:

- a demonstration through which an insurer will reimburse participating hospitals through a payment system that links patient outcomes with provider reimbursements;
- a demonstration of the extent to which an intensified program of post-hospital care for high-risk patients can improve their prospects for full, uneventful recoveries and reduce total costs per episode of illness; and
- a feasibility study of the creation of a geriatric day hospital as a cost- and outcome-effective alternative to inpatient, nursing home, and home care within the broader, interdisciplinary geriatrics program of an academic medical center.

Although the existence of problems and possible solutions to them are two prerequisites for policymaking, they do not ensure the development of policy. Public policies are made within a political context. Thus, strategymakers can also influence the policy agenda through their involvement in the political circumstances that help shape the agenda.

Political Circumstances

A variety of political circumstances help create windows of opportunity through which policy issues move to the stage at which legislation may be developed to address them (see Figure 5.1). These political circumstances include such factors as:

- the public attitudes, concerns, and opinions surrounding issues;
- the policy preferences of various individuals and interest groups, including strategymakers in healthcare organizations, and their relative ability to influence political decisions;
- the positions of key political leaders on issues; and
- the scope and complexity of competing issues on the policy agenda at any particular point.

Strategymakers have available to them two especially powerful methods of influencing the political circumstances that affect a particular policy issue. First, they can present and push their views, often through interest groups, and often in the form of lobbying (this will be described in greater detail in Chapter 6). Second, they can seek to exert their influence by filing or joining others in filing lawsuits in which they challenge existing policies, seek to stimulate new policies, or try to alter certain aspects of the implementation of policies.

Advocating viewpoints and lobbying to influence the policy agenda: In efforts to advocate their views and to lobby for their preferences, strategymakers in healthcare organizations are supported by one of the most significant features of the political economy of the United States: the existence of the concentrated interests of those who earn their livelihoods in this domain or who are positioned to gain specific advantageous benefits for the organizations they govern and manage.

One direct result of the existence of concentrated interests is the formation of organized interest groups (Miller 1985; Ornstein and Elder 1978). An interest group "is an organization of people with similar policy goals who enter the political process to try to achieve those aims" (Lineberry, Edwards, and Wattenberg 1995, 216). Interest groups can seek to influence the formulation, implementation, and modification of policies for the purpose of providing the group's members some advantage, although in this section the focus is on their role in helping to shape the policy agenda as part of the formulation phase of the policymaking process depicted in Figure 5.1.

Because all interest groups seek policies that favor their members, their agendas and behaviors are rather predictable. Feldstein (1988) argues, for example, that healthcare provider interest groups seek to accomplish through legislation such purposes as increasing the demand for members' services, limiting competitors, permitting members to charge the highest possible prices for their services, and lowering their members' operating costs as much as possible. In contrast, an interest group representing a group of consumers of healthcare services (e.g., the American Association of Retired Persons, or AARP) would seek through public policies to minimize the costs of services to members, ease their access to services, and increase the availability of services their members want.

Interest groups play powerful roles in setting the nation's health policy agenda, as they do subsequently in the development of legislation and in the implementation and modification of policies. These groups can play their roles proactively by seeking to stimulate new policies that serve the interests of their members, or they can play their roles reactively by seeking to block policy changes they do not believe serve their members' best interests. Interest groups are an inherent part of the public policymaking process in the United States. Recent decades have brought an expansion of astonishing proportions in their involvement in the policymaking process (Scholzman and Tierney 1986); these groups seem especially ubiquitous in the health sector.

All strategymakers in healthcare organizations have ready access to membership in interest groups and to the collective influence such memberships afford. Those in hospitals, for example, can join the AHA and their state hospital associations. If they prefer a collective voice more specifically focused on their policy interests, managers in teaching hospitals can link their organizations to the Council of Teaching Hospitals (COTH), those in children's hospitals can join the National Association of Children's Hospitals and Related Institutions, and those in investor-owned hospitals can align themselves with the Federation of American Health Systems (FAHS). These and many other interest groups provide their members a way to link their policy preferences into more powerful, collective voices that greatly increase the likelihood of significant impact on the policy agenda.

Examples of several ways that strategymakers, working through interest groups, have sought to influence the policy agenda are reflected in actions taken by the AHA and other interest groups in the face of congressional consideration in 1995 of possible substantial reductions in federal spending on the Medicare program. These deliberations occurred in the context of an overall effort to balance the federal budget over a seven-year span. One example is the congressional testimony given by Richard Davidson, president of the AHA, on the issue of the long-term implications of severe cuts in federal support for the Medicare program. Testifying before the Senate Finance Committee on May 17, 1995, and reported in the May 22, 1995, issue of *AHA News*, Mr. Davidson said that "On Medicare's 30th anniversary, lawmakers should think about the next 30 years, not the immediate future." His testimony included other points in support of the preferences of the AHA's membership regarding the policy agenda for the Medicare program: He said, "Spending reductions in GOP budget plans under congressional consideration would only breathe a few years of life into Medicare's ailing hospital trust fund." In this testimony, he also renewed the AHA's call for the creation of a permanent, independent citizen's commission that would try to match Congress's spending targets with the kind of benefits that such allocations would buy.

Also on May 17, 1995, the AHA and the FAHS, joined by 20 other healthcare provider interest groups, sent a letter to all members of the House of Representatives stating that, "We know that savings in the [Medicare] system can be achieved, and we are willing to accept some reductions through restructuring. The proposals put forward by the House Budget Committee, however, [which were designed to slow the growth in federal spending on the Medicare program by $283 billion over seven years] go too far, too fast." Finally, on that day, the AHA and the federation ran a series of ads in newspapers widely read by federal policymakers asking the policymakers to work with these interest groups "to reform, restructure and save money in Medicare—not gut it."

These and other related activities represented attempts by the involved interest groups to help redefine Medicare cost escalation as a long-term problem that would interfere with people getting the services they need rather than a short-term budgetary problem and to offer an alternative solution (the proposed citizen's commission) to addressing the problem. In short, they sought to influence the health policy agenda as it pertains to the Medicare program and, through this, to help shape Medicare policy. This is a vivid example of the role that interest groups play shaping the health policy agenda. More about this role and the other roles that interest groups play in the larger policymaking process will be covered in Chapter 6.

Using the courts to influence the policy agenda: The use of both state and federal courts, as a means to influence public policymaking in the health domain, is increasing. In recent years, the courts have heavily influenced the health policy agenda in four areas: the coverage decisions made by insurers in both the private and public sectors, the Medicaid program's payment rates to hospitals and nursing homes, the antitrust issues involved in hospital mergers, and issues related to the charitable mission and tax-exempt status of nonprofit hospitals (Anderson 1992; Potter and Longest 1994).

A court provides one very important structural advantage to those who seek to influence the health policy agenda: a narrow focus on the issues involved in a specific case. Strategymakers who initiate court cases have the opportunity to control, at least to a significant degree, the issues to be addressed and to have their sides of the issues receive detailed attention. This stands in stark contrast to the wide-open, if not chaotic, political arena in which most efforts to influence the policy agenda must take place.

An example of how strategymakers in healthcare organizations can use a court to influence the public policy agenda can be seen in the ruling by the U.S. Supreme Court in April 1995 that the federal Employee Retirement Income Security Act (ERISA) does not impede states from setting hospital rates. The case that resulted in this ruling arose out of New York's practice of adding a surcharge to certain hospital bills to raise money to help fund healthcare for some of the state's low-income citizens. The state's practice was challenged by the strategymakers in a group of commercial insurers, HMOs, and by New York City (Green 1995a). A number of healthcare interest groups filed a joint *amicus curiae* ("friend of the court") brief in the case in which they asserted that Congress, in enacting ERISA, never intended for it to be used to challenge state health reform plans and initiatives. The Supreme Court's ruling is seen generally as supportive of state efforts to broaden healthcare services to their poorer residents through various reforms and initiatives. In this sense, it helps broaden the potential solutions available to address the problem of providing healthcare to the nation's uninsured citizens. That is, the court's ruling in this case has helped shape the public policy agenda regarding this issue.

Strategymakers are far more likely to influence public policies, and the effects of the policies on their organizations, through state courts and lower federal courts than through their relatively rare opportunities to do so before the U.S. Supreme Court. Recent examples of this technique can be seen in courts in Pennsylvania in cases involving the tax-exempt status of healthcare organizations. In one 1995 case, the Indiana County (PA) Court of Common Pleas rebuffed the strategymakers of Indiana Hospital in their appeal to have the hospital's tax-exempt status restored after the exemption had been revoked by the county in 1993. In making its ruling, the court held that the hospital failed to meet one of the state's tests adequately through which an organization qualifies for tax exemption. Among other rules, the state requires a tax-exempt organization "to donate or render gratuitously a substantial portion of its services."

In so ruling, the Indiana County Court took note of the fact that Indiana Hospital's uncompensated charity care in fiscal year 1994 had been approximately two percent of its total expected compensation and contrasted this with an earlier case resulting from the revocation of the tax-exempt status of a nursing home in the state. The state Supreme Court decision in the St. Margaret Seneca Place nursing home case had been that the nursing home did meet the state's test because it demonstrated that it bore more than one-third of the cost of care for half its patients. The variation in these and several other Pennsylvania cases in the courts' interpretation of the meaning of the state's partial test for tax-exempt status (i.e., the requirement that a tax-exempt organization is "to donate or render gratuitously a substantial portion of its services") has led a coalition of tax-exempt organizations in the state to seek clarifying legislation on this and other points regarding the determination of tax-exempt status. As a result of their efforts, Senate Bill 355, the Institutions of Purely Public Charity Act, has been introduced in the Pennsylvania legislature.

Exerting Influence in the Development of Legislation

Once health policy issues achieve prominence on the policy agenda, they can proceed to the next stage of the policy formulation phase— development of legislation (see Figure 5.1). At this stage, specific legislative proposals go through a process involving a carefully prescribed set of steps (described in Chapter 3) that can, but do not always, lead to policies in the form of new legislation, or as is more often the case, amendments to previously enacted legislation. In fact, only a small fraction of policy issues result in the development of specific legislation that is intended to address the issues. And even then, only some of the attempts to enact legislation are successful. While the path for legislation is indeed long and arduous, it is replete with opportunities for strategymakers to influence legislation development.

Both as individuals and through the interest groups to which they belong, strategymakers participate directly in actually drafting legislative proposals and frequently participate in the hearings associated with the development of legislation. An example of this latter technique for influencing the development of legislation can be found in the consideration by the Pennsylvania legislature in 1995 of so-called "any willing provider" legislation.

As part of the legislation development process, the Pennsylvania House of Representatives Insurance Committee held a series of hearings in 1995 on the potential legislation, House Bill 630. This bill would have created a circumstance in which managed care networks and health plans would have found it much more difficult to exclude providers from their networks, thus reducing their ability to contract selectively for the utilization of the services of providers whom they judged to be acceptably efficient in their professional practice and who met their quality standards. Healthcare strategymakers' concerns about such legislation were intense at the time of these hearings, both in Pennsylvania and across the nation. In fact, grouping their concerns about any willing provider laws with their concerns about mandatory point of service laws into a broader set of concerns they refer to as "selective contracting restrictions," the strategymakers in the nation's managed care plans identified such restrictions as the top item on their public policy agenda for 1995 (Ernst & Young 1995).

At the first of four hearings in the series, which was sponsored by the Pennsylvania House of Representatives Insurance Committee, a strategymaker from one of Pennsylvania's larger healthcare systems, representing the Hospital Association of Pennsylvania, testified that the proposed legislation was anti-competitive in that it would "destroy the gatekeeper concept that is central to managed care, severely limiting a managed care organization's ability to control health care costs and the quality of their networks" (Hospital Association of Pennsylvania 1995, 2).

Strategymakers or their spokespersons from several other organizations and healthcare interest groups also testified at this hearing in an effort to influence the development of this legislation, including Blue Cross of Northeastern Pennsylvania, the Insurance Federation of Pennsylvania, Pennsylvania Nurses Association, Geisinger Health Plan, and HealthAmerica (an HMO). The views on this legislation of the Patient Advocacy Coalition, several individual physicians, and a pharmacist were also presented at this hearing.

Influencing Rulemaking

Enacted legislation rarely contains enough explicit language to guide its implementation completely. Rather, laws are often vague on implementation details, leaving the implementing agencies and organizations to establish the rules and regulations needed to put the legislation into operation. The promulgation of rules, as a formal part of the implementation phase, is guided by certain rules. Key among these at the federal level, with parallels in most of the states, is the requirement that the organization responsible for implementing a law (e.g., the HCFA) publish an NPRM in the *Federal Register*. A NPRM is, in effect, a draft of a rule or set of rules under development. Publication of this notice is an open invitation to those with an interest in the rules and regulations applicable to implementing a particular policy to react to proposed or draft rules before they become final.

The procedure of commenting on draft rules is one of the most active points of involvement for the strategymakers for healthcare organizations and others who have a stake in a particular policy in the entire policymaking process. This point of involvement can produce significant results. Changes in proposed rules often result from what Thompson (1991, 149) calls the "strategic interaction" that occurs between implementing organizations and those affected by their rules during rulemaking. For example, among the numerous rules proposed in implementing the 1974 National Health Planning and Resources Development Act (P.L. 93-641) were some that sought to reduce obstetrical capacity in the nation's hospitals. One proposed rule, in 1977, called for hospitals to perform at least 500 deliveries annually or close their obstetrical units. Notice of this proposed rule elicited immediate and vigorous objections, especially from the strategymakers from hospitals in rural areas where obstetrical care was needed but where meeting the rule's threshold of 500 deliveries annually could be difficult or impossible. As a result, the final rules were far less restrictive, in fact making no reference at all to a specific number of deliveries that hospitals in rural areas should perform (Zwick 1978).

A more recent example of the ability of strategymakers from healthcare organizations to influence public policymaking through influence on rulemaking can be seen in an apparent change in the way the FTC plans to interpret certain rules in antitrust cases involving hospitals. Historically, the FTC focused on product and geographic markets and on competitive effects in their antitrust enforcement efforts aimed at hospital mergers. It has not viewed efficiency as a major factor in its analyses of possible hospital mergers. Now, however, following a long period during which healthcare strategymakers, working through their interest groups and through arguments presented in antitrust cases involving hospital mergers, have argued that improved efficiencies gained through mergers are an extremely important means of helping to contain healthcare costs, it appears that these views have affected the FTC. A reported account of a public speech given by FTC Commissioner Christine Varney in Chicago on May 2, 1995, states that she discussed plans whereby

> the agency is abandoning its "linear" method to hospital-merger antitrust enforcement for a more "holistic" approach that accommodates the field's peculiarities.
>
> Varney said this uniqueness, paired with the special nature of hospital-merger analysis, "virtually mandates that antitrust enforcers carefully examine asserted efficiencies before determining whether to challenge a particular hospital merger."
>
> From now on, Varney said, improved hospital efficiency resulting from mergers will be presumed to benefit consumers when mergers do not threaten competition (Green 1995b).

In addition to exerting their influence directly by commenting on the rules that will guide the implementation of policies, strategymakers can also use two other means to influence policymaking at this stage. When the development of rules and regulations is anticipated to be unusually difficult or contentious, or when rules and regulations are anticipated to be subject to continuous revision, special task forces may be established to help with their development. For example, after passage of the Health Maintenance Organization Act (P.L. 9–227) in 1973, the Department of Health, Education, and Welfare (DHEW) (now DHHS) organized a series of task forces, including on them some people who were or would become strategymakers in this industry, to help develop the proposed rules for implementing the law. This approach, which involved strategymakers in the development of rules, produced rules that were much more acceptable to those who would be affected by them than might otherwise have been the case.

Another approach to support rulemaking is the creation of advisory commissions to assist with the ongoing rulemaking effort directly. This, too, provides a means through which strategymakers can exert their influence. For example, following enactment of the 1983 Amendments to the Social Security Act (P.L. 98-21), which established the PPS for reimbursing hospitals for the care of Medicare beneficiaries, Congress established ProPAC to provide nonbinding advice to the HCFA in implementing the reimbursement system. Later, a second commission, the PPRC, was established to advise Congress and HCFA regarding payment for physicians' services under the Medicare program. These commissions have been useful in helping HCFA to make required annual decisions regarding reimbursement rates, fees, and other variables in the operation of the Medicare program.

Although the opportunities for direct service on such commissions are limited to very few people, others can influence their thinking. Strategymakers can seek to influence the thinking of commission members, and thus the advice commission members ultimately provide to Congress and to HCFA, by sharing their ideas, experiences, and data as inputs to commission deliberations.

Influencing Policymaking at the Stage of Policy Operation

The policy operation stage of implementing policies involves the actual running of programs and activities embedded in or stimulated by enacted legislation. Operation is the responsibility, primarily, of the appointees and civil servants who staff the government, and who influence policies by their operational decisions and actions made in implementing them. Thus, strategymakers can influence policies by influencing those who manage the operation of policies. This form of influence arises from the working relationships that can be developed between those responsible for implementing public policies and those whom their decisions and activities directly effect, such as the strategymakers in healthcare organizations.

The opportunities to build these relationships are supported by a prominent feature of the careers of bureaucrats—longevity (Kingdon 1995). Elected policymakers come and go, but the bureaucracy endures. Strategymakers, and other participants in their healthcare organizations, can and do build long-standing working relationships with some of the people responsible for implementing the public policies that are of strategic importance to these organizations.

The most solid base for these working relationships is the exchange of useful information and expertise. A strategymaker, speaking from an authoritative position based on actual operational experience with the implementation of a policy, can influence the policy's further implementation with relevant information. If the information supports change, especially if it buttressed with similar information from others who are experiencing the effect of a particular policy, reasonable implementors may well be influenced to make needed changes. This is especially likely if there is a well-established working relationship based on mutual respect for the roles of and the challenges facing each party.

Sometimes the relationships between strategymakers in healthcare organizations, usually operating through their interest groups, and those responsible for implementing policies important to them are expanded to include members of the legislative committees or subcommittees with jurisdiction over the policies. This triad of mutual interests forms what has been termed an *iron triangle*, so called because the interests of the three parts of the triangle "dovetail nicely and because they are alleged to be impenetrable from the outside and uncontrollable by president, political appointees, or legislators not on the committees in question" (Kingdon 1995, 33).

The enormity of the bureaucracy with which they might need to interact is an obvious and very limiting problem for strategymakers wishing to influence the policymaking process though influencing either the rulemaking or policy operation stages of policy implementation. Consider how many components of the federal government are involved in rulemaking and policy operation that is directly relevant to healthcare organizations. Add to this the units of state and local government that are relevant and the challenge of keeping track of where working relationships might be useful as a means of influencing policymaking—to say nothing of actually developing and maintaining the relationships—

and the magnitude of the process becomes clear. Obviously, selectivity in which of these relationships might be of most strategic importance, as well as reliance upon the interest groups to which they belong to do much of the relationship building, helps strategymakers face such a daunting challenge.

Exerting Influence Through Policy Modification

Policy modification occurs when the outcomes, perceptions, and consequences of existing policies feed back into the agenda-setting and legislation development stages of the formulation phase and into the rulemaking and policy operation stages of the implementation phase and stimulate changes in legislation, rules, or operations (see the feedback loop running along the bottom of Figure 5.1). Although some health policies are developed *de novo*, as was noted in Chapter 3, the vast majority of them result from the modification of existing policies in rather modest, incremental steps.

Following the feedback loop shown in Figure 5.1, it can be seen that because agenda setting involves the confluence of problems, possible solutions, and political circumstances, policy modification can occur at this stage in a number of ways. As problems become more sharply defined and better understood through the actual experiences of those who are affected by the policies, modifications can be triggered. Strategymakers and others involved in healthcare organizations are the best sources of feedback on the consequences of policies for their organizations and, in some cases, the populations they serve. Similarly, possible new solutions to problems can be conceived and assessed through the operational experiences of strategymakers with particular policies, and, especially, when the results of demonstrations and evaluations provide concrete evidence of the performance of particular solutions that are under consideration. Finally, the interactions among the branches of government and strategymakers and their interest groups who are involved with and affected by ongoing policies become important components of the political circumstances surrounding the amendment of these policies.

The outcomes, perceptions, and consequences that flow from the ongoing policymaking process also help modify policies by directly influencing the development of legislation. Actual experience with the effect of the implementation of policies that affect their organizations help strategymakers to identify routinely needed modifications to such policies. The history of the Medicare program is a good example of this phenomenon. Over the program's life, services have been added and deleted; premiums and copayment provisions have been changed; reimbursement mechanisms have been changed; features to ensure quality and medical necessity of services have been added, changed, and deleted; and so on. The inputs of strategymakers from healthcare organizations, based upon their experiences with Medicare policy, played a role in each of these amendments to the original legislation, although other influences also helped guide these changes.

Strategymakers also have extensive opportunities to influence the modification of policies in their implementation phases, in both the rulemaking and policy operation stages. The modification of rules, as well as changes in the operations undertaken to implement policies, often reflect the actual reported or documented experiences of those affected by the rules and operations. Strategymakers can provide this feedback directly to those with rulemaking or operational responsibilities. They can also take their views on the rules and operational practices that affect their organizations to the courts or the legislative branch. Both can also be pathways to modifications.

The implementation of the Occupational Safety and Health Act (P.L. 91-596) in 1970 illustrates well how readily the strategymakers in health-care organizations, as well as in many other types of organizations, can use the courts to influence rules and operational practices (Robinson and Paxman 1991). This legislation set in motion a massive federal program of standard setting and enforcement that sought to improve safety and health conditions in the nation's workplaces. As Thompson (1981) has noted, managers and labor leaders "have repeatedly appealed decisions by the Occupational Safety and Health Administration (OSHA) to the courts. The development of this program in some respects reads like a legal history" (24).

Similarly, the rules promulgated to implement the Medicare and Medicaid legislation, as well as the operational decisions and actions of HCFA as the implementing organization, have frequently been challenged in the courts. Public policies of relevance to the strategymakers in healthcare organizations in such diverse areas as human resources, clinical laboratories, and mergers and acquisitions have also been challenged in court.

As demonstrated by the examples given above, there are abundant opportunities for strategymakers to influence public policymaking. Their influence can be exerted in both the agenda-setting and legislation development stages of the formulation phase and in both the rulemaking and policy operation stages of the implementation phase of the policymaking process. Furthermore, there are continuing opportunities for influencing policies as the outcomes, perceptions, and consequences that result from them trigger policy modification. In effect, those who would influence policies have an opportunity to do so in the initial iteration of the process in regard to any particular policy, but they also get additional opportunities to exert their influence through the subsequent modification of existing policies. The multiple opportunities for strategymakers to influence public policymaking are summarized in Figure 5.2.

In addition to having a number of places in the policymaking process to exert influence, strategymakers have three sources of power available to them in their influence activities: positional, capacity to reward or coerce, and expertise. Figure 5-3 combines the places where influence can be exerted within the policymaking process with the sources of power that can be used in exerting influence to illustrate in summary fashion the great variety of opportunities available to strategymakers to influence their organization's public policy environment.

The numerous opportunities that strategymakers in healthcare organizations have to influence policy and the variety of influence mechanisms described in this chapter, however, say little about the actual manner in which such influence can or should be exerted. The code of ethics of the American College of Healthcare Executives (ACHE) provides some guidance for strategymakers in their efforts to influence public policymaking by stating that they should "participate in public dialogue on healthcare policy issues and advocate solutions that will improve health status and promote quality healthcare" (American College

Figure 5.2 Opportunities for Strategymakers to Influence Policymaking

I. Influencing Policy Formulation
    A. Agenda Setting
        1. Defining and documenting problems
        2. Developing and evaluating solutions
        3. Shaping political circumstances through lobbying and the courts
    B. Legislation Development
        1. Participating in drafting legislation
        2. Testifying at legislative hearings
II. Influencing Policy Implementation
    A. Rulemaking
        1. Providing formal comments on draft rules
        2. Serving on and providing input to rulemaking advisory bodies
    B. Policy Operation
        1. Interactions with policy operators
III. Influencing Policy Modification
    A. Documenting the case for modification through operational experience and formal evaluations

Figure 5.3 The Opportunities to Exert Influence in Public Policy Environments

	Problem Definition	Identifying Solutions	Political Circumstances	Legislation Development	Rulemaking	Policy Operation
Power Based on Position						
Power to Reward/Coerce						
Power Based on Expertise						

of Healthcare Executives 1994: Section IV, C). But more needs to be said about the ethics of influencing public policy. There is an abiding danger that these activities can involve unethical behavior.

Ethical Considerations in Influencing Policy

Ethics play an important part in public policymaking, albeit only a part. Ethical principles can provide the moral background for a health policy, but in addition, "the policy itself must be informed by empirical data and by special information available in the fields of medicine, biology, law, psychology, and so on" (Beauchamp and Childress 1989: 14).

Ethical behavior, for any and all participants in policymaking (including strategymakers who seek to influence policy), can be guided in important ways by four philosophical principles: respect for the autonomy of others, justice, beneficence, and nonmaleficence. Each of these is considered below, beginning with the concept of respect for autonomy. This concept is based on the notion that individuals have the right to their own beliefs and values and to the decisions and choices that further these beliefs and values. Regarding healthcare, where respect for the autonomy of other people is of extreme importance, this principle pertains to the rights of individuals to independent self-determination regarding how they live their lives and to their rights regarding the integrity of their bodies and minds.

Respect for autonomy is important in such contemporary health policy considerations as those involving privacy and individual choice, including behavioral or lifestyle choices. Policies that do not reflect a respect for the autonomy of others are paternalistic. One vivid example of the kind of policies that result from adherence to the principle of autonomy in health policymaking is the 1990 Patient Self-Determination

Act. This policy was designed to facilitate the efforts of people to exercise their right to make decisions concerning their medical care, including the right to accept or refuse treatment, and the right to formulate advance directives regarding their care. Strategymakers, and others, who supported this policy were acting in a manner consistent with respect for the autonomy of others.

The principle of respect for autonomy includes several other elements that are especially important in guiding ethical behavior in those who influence policymaking. One of these is honesty: telling the truth. Respect for people as autonomous beings implies honesty in relationships with them. The element of confidentiality is closely related to honesty in such relationships. Confidences broken in the policymaking process can impair the process. A third element of the autonomy principle with relevance to the policymaking process is fidelity. This means doing one's duty and keeping one's word, which is often equated with promise keeping. When strategymakers who seek to influence policy tell the truth, honor confidences, and keep promises, their behavior is more ethically sound than if these things are not done.

Justice is a second ethical principle of significant importance to those who influence policymaking. The practical implications for public policymaking of the principle of justice are felt mostly in terms of distributive justice; that is, in terms of fairness in the distribution of healthcare benefits and burdens in society. Attention to the ethical principle of justice, of course, raises the question of what is fair. Allocative policies that adhere closely to the principle of justice allocate burdens and benefits according to the provisions of a morally defensible system rather than through arbitrary or capricious decisions. Regulatory policies guided by the principle of justice fairly and equitably affect those to whom the regulations are targeted.

Two other ethical principles have direct relevance to policymaking and to efforts by strategymakers to influence this process: beneficence and nonmaleficence. Beneficence in policymaking means acting with charity and kindness. This principle is incorporated into acts through which benefits are provided, and thus beneficence characterizes most allocative policies. But beneficence also includes the more complex concept of balancing benefits and harms, for using the relative costs and benefits of alternative decisions and actions as one basis upon which to choose from among alternatives. The growing emphasis on cost-effectiveness in healthcare and the development of policies to achieve this goal will increasingly call into play the principle of beneficence in developing ethically sound policies. Strategymakers will be in danger of violating this principle of ethical behavior when they seek policies that exclusively serve the interests of their organizations rather than maximizing the net benefits to society as a whole.

Nonmaleficence, a principle with deep roots in medical ethics, is exemplified in the dictum *primum non nocere*—first, do no harm. When strategymakers who influence policy are guided by this principle, they seek to minimize harm to society as a whole. The principles of beneficence and nonmaleficence are clearly reflected in health policies that ensure the quality of healthcare services and products. Such policies as those establishing Professional Review Organizations (PROs) to review the quality of care provided to Medicare patients and the policies that the FDA uses to ensure the safety of pharmaceuticals are examples. Policies that support the conduct and use of outcome studies of clinical care are also examples.

Although adherence to the principles of respect for the autonomy of other people, justice, beneficence, and nonmaleficence does not ensure that policies supported by strategymakers necessarily are in the best strategic interests of their organizations, such adherence does place the strategymakers on relatively high ethical ground.

Summary

The public policies that are relevant to healthcare organizations are made through a highly complex, interactive, and cyclical process that incorporates formulation, implementation, and modification phases of activities. (The public policymaking process is described in detail in Chapter 3.) The process is played out in the context of a political marketplace with diverse participants. Participants include elected and appointed members of all three branches of government as well as civil servants who staff the government on the one hand, and strategymakers and others whose organizations are affected by policies or who are personally affected by policies, and the interest groups to which they belong, on the other hand. The policymaking process includes a number of opportunities for the latter group of participants to influence the policies made by the former group.

In this chapter, the model of the public policymaking process has been used to provide a map to the places in the process where strategymakers can exert their influence (see Figure 5.1). In the agenda-setting stage of policy formulation, strategymakers can help define the problems that policies might address, they can participate in designing possible solutions to them, and they can help create the political circumstances necessary to advance the potential solutions to actual policies. Their central roles in the health sector equip the strategymakers of healthcare organizations to be well informed about certain kinds of healthcare problems that should be addressed through public policies. The resources at their command and their abilities to permit their organizations to serve as demonstration sites for assessing possible solutions facilitate their roles in identifying feasible solutions to problems. And their abilities, as individuals and through interest groups, to lobby for their preferences and to use the courts as allies in seeking to have their policy preferences enacted provide effective mechanisms through which these strategymakers can participate in shaping the political circumstances surrounding a policy issue.

Strategymakers can also exert influence on policymaking in the legislation development stage of the process. Here, again acting both as individuals and through their interest groups, they can participate in the actual drafting of legislative proposals and they can provide testimony in the hearings in which legislation is developed.

Rulemaking, procedurally, is designed to include input from those who will be affected by the rules, such as strategymakers in the health sector. This input can be made through formal comment on proposed rules. Influence can also be exerted through inputs to task forces and commissions established by rulemaking agencies as a means to obtain advice on their work. In the policy operation stage, strategymakers can influence policies by influencing those with policy operation responsibilities. This is done best through establishing and maintaining effective working relationships with members of the implementing bureaucracy.

This chapter notes that strategymakers can exert their influence in the initial iterations of the process through which policies are made. But, importantly, because policymaking is a cyclical process in which the results of policies continuously feed back into the process where they trigger modifications, there are subsequent opportunities to influence policies—again in the agenda-setting, legislation development, rulemaking, and policy operation stages of the process. In effect, strategymakers have multiple opportunities to influence policymaking and resultant policies.

Given the importance of public policies to the strategic success of healthcare organizations, their strategymakers should avail themselves of the many opportunities to influence relevant policies that are described in this chapter. However, their efforts should be guided by ethical considerations. Four principles that can be useful in guiding strategymakers to more ethical policy-influencing behaviors and activities are respect for the autonomy of other people, justice, beneficence, and nonmaleficence.

References

American College of Healthcare Executives. *Code of Ethics*. Chicago: American College of Healthcare Executives. As Amended on August 9, 1994.

Anderson, G. F. 1992. "The Courts and Health Policy: Strengths and Limitations." *Health Affairs* 11 (Fall): 95–110.

Beauchamp, T. L., and J. F. Childress. 1989. *Principles of Biomedical Ethics*, 3rd ed. New York: Oxford University Press.

Buchholz, R. 1989. *Environments and Public Policy*. Englewood Cliffs, NJ: Prentice Hall.

———. 1993. *Management Response to Public Issues*, 3rd ed. Englewood Cliffs, NJ: Prentice Hall.

Cerne, F. 1993. "Hospital Cooperation Act Opens Door to Increased Collaboration." *Hospitals* 67 (5): 27.

Ernst & Young LLP. 1995. "Anti-Selective Contracting Laws." *CapitolWATCH* 95(5): 2.

Evans, R. G., and G. L. Stoddart. 1994. "Producing Health, Consuming Health Care," 27–64. In *Why Are Some People Healthy and Others Not? The Determinants of Health of Populations*, edited by R. G. Evans, M. L. Barer, and T. R. Marmor. New York: Aldine De Gruyter.

Feldstein, P. J. 1988. *The Politics of Health Legislation: An Economic Perspective*. Ann Arbor, MI: Health Administration Press.

Green, J. 1995a. "High-Court Ruling Protects Hospital-bill Surcharges." *AHA News* 31 (18): 1.

———. 1995b. "FTC Ruling Clears Way for Hospital Mergers." *AHA News* 31 (19): 1.

Hospital Association of Pennsylvania. 1995. "HAP Testifies Any Willing Provider Legislation Can Do More Harm Than Good." *Pennsylvania Hospitals Nineties* 6 (10): 1.

Kania, A. J. 1993. "Legislation Gives Maine Hospitals OK for Collaboration." *Health Care Strategic Management* 11 (5): 12–13.

Keys, B., and T. Case. 1990. "How to Become an Influential Manager." *The Executive* 4 (November): 38–51.

Kingdon, J. W. 1995. *Agendas, Alternatives, and Public Policies*, 2nd ed. Boston: Little, Brown & Company.

Lineberry, R. T., G. C. Edwards, III, and M. P. Wattenberg. 1995. *Government in America: People, Politics, and Policy*, Brief Version, 2nd ed. New York: HarperCollins College Publishers.

Longest, B. B., Jr. 1988. "American Health Policy in the Year 2000." *Hospital & Health Services Administration* 33 (4): 419–34.

———. 1994. *Health Policymaking in the United States*. Ann Arbor, MI: Health Administration Press.

Michaud, S. R. "Breaking New Ground: Antitrust Policy and Health Care Provider Coalitions." A public lecture in the Lecture Series in Health Management and Policy sponsored by the Health Policy Institute at the University of Pittsburgh, October 20, 1992.

Miller, S. 1985. *Special Interest Groups in American Politics*. New Brunswick, NJ: Transaction Books.

Mintzberg, H. 1983. *Power In and Around Organizations.* Englewood Cliffs, NJ: Prentice Hall.

Morlock, L. L., C. A. Nathanson, and J. A. Alexander. 1988. "Authority, Power, and Influence." 265–300. In *Health Care Management: A Text in Organization Theory and Behavior*, 2nd ed., edited by S. M. Shortell and A. D. Kaluzny. New York: John Wiley & Sons.

Ornstein, N., and S. Elder. 1978. *Interest Groups, Lobbying and Policymaking.* Washington, DC: Congressional Quarterly Press.

Potter, M. A., and B. B. Longest, Jr. 1994. "The Divergence of Federal and State Policies on the Charitable Tax Exemption of Nonprofit Hospitals." *Journal of Health Politics, Policy and Law* 19 (Summer): 393–419.

Robinson, J. C., and D. G. Paxman. 1991. "Technological, Economic, and Political Feasibility in OSHA's Air Contaminants Standards." *Journal of Health Politics, Policy and Law* 16 (Spring): 1–18.

Scholzman, K. L., and J. T. Tierney. 1986. *Organized Interests and American Democracy.* New York: Harper & Row.

Shortell, S. M., and U. E. Reinhardt, eds. 1992. *Improving Health Policy and Management: Nine Critical Research Issues for the 1990s.* Ann Arbor, MI: AHSR/Health Administration Press.

Thompson, F. J. 1981. *Health Policy and the Bureaucracy: Politics and Implementation.* Cambridge, MA: Massachusetts Institute of Technology Press.

———. 1991. "The Enduring Challenge of Health Policy Implementation." 148–69. In *Health Politics and Policy*, 2nd ed., edited by T. J. Litman and L. S. Robins. Albany, NY: Delmar Publishers Inc.

Zwick, D. I. 1978. "Initial Development of Guidelines for Health Planning." *Public Health Reports* 93 (5): 407–20.

6

Healthcare Interest Groups and
Their Influence on Public Policy

As was discussed in previous chapters, strategymakers in healthcare organizations face significant challenges in meeting their dual responsibilities for analyzing and influencing the public policy environments of their organizations. In their efforts to cope with the extensive and dynamic set of forces and actors at work in their public policy environments, they can turn for assistance to outside resources. Principally, they can seek assistance from the interest groups to which the strategymakers and their organizations can belong.

Strategymakers in healthcare organizations can be supported in their efforts to analyze and—especially—to influence the public policy environments of their organizations in important ways by the opportunity to join and obtain certain benefits from membership in interest groups. The role of interest groups in helping strategymakers influence these environments was introduced in the previous chapter and is expanded upon here. The discussion is extended to provide a broader background on the role of interest groups in the American public policymaking process. Readers should also gain more insight into the ways that interest groups can help strategymakers to better analyze and discern strategically important information in, and to exert influence on, the public policy environments of their organizations. Consideration of interest groups begins with an examination of two polar perspectives on the roles of such groups in public policymaking.

Two Perspectives on Interest Groups in American Policymaking

Recall from the previous chapter that an interest group is "an organization of people with similar policy goals who enter the political process to try to achieve those aims" (Lineberry, Edwards, and Wattenberg 1995, 216). Interest groups arise from the existence in democratic societies of the interests that groups of people have in particular benefits to be derived or outcomes to be achieved through their collective action within the public policymaking process. They are as ubiquitous in the United States in the healthcare domain as much as in any other. Recent decades, in fact, have brought an expansion of astonishing proportions in their involvement in the policymaking process (Scholzman and Tierney 1986).

The rights to organize such groups, as well as to participate in them, are granted and protected by the U.S. Constitution. The Constitution's First Amendment guarantees the American people the right "peaceably to assemble, and to petition the Government for a redress of grievances." However, constitutional guarantees notwithstanding, political theorists have disagreed about whether interest groups play essentially positive or negative roles in American political life since the nation's beginnings to the present day (Bauer, Pool, and Dexter 1963; Olson 1965; Truman 1971; Wilson 1973; Ornstein and Elder 1978; Moe 1980; Peters 1986; Morone 1990; Lineberry, Edwards, and Wattenberg 1995).

James Madison, writing in several of *The Federalist Papers* in 1788, discussed the relationship of groups, which he called "factions," to democratic government. In *Federalist* Number 10, he defined a faction as "a number of citizens, whether amounting to a majority or a minority of the whole, who are united and actuated by some common impulse of passion, or of interest, adverse to the rights of citizens, or to the permanent and aggregate interests of the community." As can be seen in the last part of his definition, Madison felt strongly that factions, or interest groups, were inherently bad. He also believed, however, that the formation of such groups was a natural outgrowth of human nature (he wrote in *Federalist* Number 10 that "the latent causes of faction are sown into the nature of man") and that government should not seek to check this activity. In his wisdom, Madison felt that what he called the "mischiefs of faction" could and should be contained by setting the "ambition" of one faction against the selfish preferences and behaviors of other factions or groups. So began an enduring history of uncertainty about and ambiguity toward the role of interest groups in public policymaking in the United States. One point about which there is neither uncertainty nor ambiguity is that interest groups play active roles in the public policymaking process.

Reflecting widely divergent views on the manner in which interest groups play their roles in the public policymaking process, two very distinct theories or models of how groups influence policymaking have emerged: the pluralist and the elitist models. Each model is examined in turn below.

The Pluralist Perspective

Some believe that because there are so many interest groups everyone's interests can be represented by one or more of them. This is the pluralist perspective on the role of interest groups in policymaking. Adherents to the pluralist model usually believe that interest groups play essentially positive roles in public policymaking. The pluralists argue that a large variety of interest groups compete with and counterbalance each other in the political marketplace where public policymaking occurs.

Adherents to the pluralist perspective do not question that some groups are stronger than others, nor do they generally doubt that competing interests do not necessarily get equal hearings. However, pluralists argue that power is widely dispersed among competing groups, with groups winning some of the time and losing some of the time in getting their preferred outcomes.

Pluralist theory about how the policymaking process works includes several interconnected arguments that, when taken together, constitute what has come to be called a group theory of politics (Truman 1971). The central tenets of the group theory of how the public policymaking process works, at all levels of government, include the following:

- Interest groups provide essential links between people and their government.
- Interest groups compete among themselves for outcomes of the policymaking process, with the interests of some groups counterbalanced by the interests of others.
- No group is likely to become too dominant; as groups become powerful, other countervailing interests organize or existing groups intensify their efforts. An important mechanism for maintaining balance among the competing groups is their ability to rely upon various sources of power; groups representing concentrated economic interests may have money, but consumer groups may have larger numbers of members.
- The competition among interest groups is basically fair. Although there are exceptions, groups typically play by the rules of the game.

In the face of a large and growing number of interest groups, some observers have concluded that the pluralist approach of encouraging and facilitating the formation of interest groups is out of control. Indeed, a large number of groups have emerged to play parts in the American policymaking process. There are more than 23,000 nonprofit interest groups with national memberships in such fields as business, education, religion, science, and healthcare in the United States today actively pursuing a variety of policy interests on behalf of their members (*Encyclopedia of Associations* 1993). The problem according to the critics of pluralism, is not merely the large number of groups, but the fact that government seems to consider the demands and preferences of all interest groups to be legitimate and seeks to somehow advance them all simultaneously.

There is little argument that government does indeed attempt to satisfy the preferences of many interests, sometimes in conflicting ways. Lowi (1979) coined the phrase "interest group liberalism" to refer to what he considers to be the federal government's excessive deference to interest groups. Others call the phenomenon *hyperpluralism* (Lineberry, Edwards, and Wattenberg 1995).

Whether they call it interest group liberalism or hyperpluralism, critics of the pluralist approach to the role of interest groups in the public policymaking process agree on two essential points:

- Interest groups have become too influential in the policymaking process; satisfying their multiple and often conflicting demands seems to drive government rather than government being driven by a desire to base policy decisions on considerations of what is best for the nation as a whole—that is, on the public interest.
- Seeking to satisfy the multiple and often conflicting demands of various interest groups leads to confusion, contradiction, and even paralysis in the policymaking process; rather than making a difficult choice between X or Y, government pretends there is no need to make the choice and seeks to satisfy both X and Y.

In addition to those who criticize the pluralist approach as being out of control and dysfunctional, there are others who believe that the perspective itself is misguided, even wrong. Instead of everyone having a chance to influence the policymaking process through one group or another, some people believe that such influence actually resides only in the hands of an elite few.

The Elitist Perspective

Whereas pluralists point with pride to how many organized interest groups actively and aggressively participate in the American process of public policymaking, people holding an elitist perspective like to point out how relatively powerless and ineffectual most of the groups are. The elitist perspective on the role of interest groups, which is quite the opposite of the pluralist viewpoint, grows out of a power-elite model of American society.

This model is based on the idea that real political power in the United States is concentrated in the hands of a very small proportion of the population that controls the nation's key institutions and organizations and much of its wealth. In the elitist perspective, these so-called "big interests" look out for themselves, in part by disproportionately influencing, if not controlling, the public policymaking process. Whether this model is an accurate reflection of how the American political system operates is debatable, but the model does indeed represent the opinions of a growing majority of Americans about who within the society has the most influence with the federal government (see Figure 6.1).

The elitist theory holds that a power elite, also referred to as the establishment, acts as a gatekeeper to the public policymaking process. That is, unless the power elite considers an issue to be important, the issue does not even get on the policy agenda. Furthermore, the theory holds

Figure 6.1   Perceptions of the Dominance of Big Interests

Question:

Would you say the government is pretty much run by a few big interests looking out for themselves or that it is run for the benefit of all the people? (The question is taken directly from National Election Studies conducted by the University of Michigan.)

Responses:

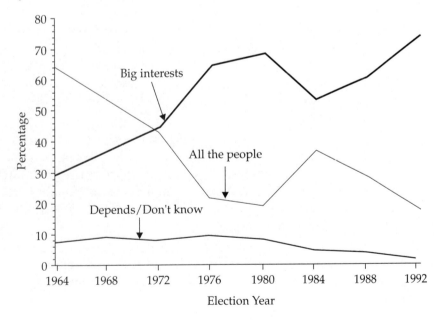

Source: *Government in America, Brief Version*, 2nd ed. (p. 219). 1995 by R. L. Lineberry, G. C. Edwards, III, and M. P. Wattenberg. New York: Reprinted with permission of HarperCollins College Publishers.

that once an issue is on the agenda, public policies made in response to triggering problems mostly reflect the values, ideologies, and preferences of this governing elite (Buchholz 1989). Thus, the power elite in society dominates public policymaking through its superior positions in society. It shapes the formulation of policies and controls their implementation through its members' powerful roles in the nation's economy and social system. It has been said that "the stability of the system, even its survival, depends upon elite consensus in behalf of the fundamental values of the system, and only policy alternatives that fall within the shared consensus will be given serious consideration" (Dye 1995, 30).

The central tenets of the power-elite theory of how the public policymaking process works in regard to the role of interest groups, which stand in stark contrast to the tenets of the group theory posited by those who hold a pluralist perspective on the process as listed above, include the following (Dye and Zeigler 1975; Lineberry, Edwards, and Wattenberg 1995):

- Real political power resides in a very small number of groups; the large number of interest groups is practically meaningless because the power differentials among them is so great. Other groups may win minor policy victories, but the power elite always prevails on the significant policy issues.

- Members of the power elite share a consensus or near-consensus on the basic values that should guide public policymaking; these values feature private property rights, the preeminence of markets and private enterprise as the best way to organize the economy, limited government, and the importance of both individual liberty and individualism.

- Members of the power elite have a strong preference for incremental changes in public policies; incrementalism in policymaking permits time for the economic and social systems to adjust to changes without these systems being threatened by them and with a minimum of economic dislocation or disruption and with minimal alteration in the social system's status quo.

- Elites protect their power bases very carefully; some limited movement of non-elites into elite positions is permitted in order to maintain social stability, but only after non-elites clearly accept the elites' consensus values.

Which Perspective Is Correct?

Those who hold the power elitist perspective challenge those who hold the pluralist perspective by pointing to the highly concentrated and interlocked power centers in American society. Studies of the concentration of political power have found that about one-third of the top leadership positions in America—corporate, foundation, and university governing boards, for example—are held by people who occupy more than one such position (Dye 1990).

Those who prefer the pluralist perspective, however, are equally quick to point to numerous examples in which those who have traditionally been grossly under-represented in the inner circles of the power elite have succeeded in collective efforts to influence significantly the public policymaking process in the United States. African Americans and women provide powerful examples of the ability of the disenfranchised—people who have long been ignored by policymakers—to organize as very effective interest groups and once so organized to redirect the course of the public policymaking process in dramatic ways.

Neither the pluralist nor the elitist perspectives alone explain how the interests of individuals, acting through their interest groups, relate to the public policymaking process. Everyone's interests are affected by the process in different degrees. Many if not all interests can influence the policymaking process, although not to equal degrees (Bibfeldt 1958). Both approaches have something of value to contribute to the thinking of strategymakers in healthcare organizations about the roles that interest groups might play in their efforts to both discern and influence the public policy environments of their organizations. At the very least, interest groups provide strategymakers with an opportunity to join with people with similar and compatible interests. In a cold, cruel world, this feature alone can be of some value. However, the potential value of interest groups goes far beyond this.

Interest groups play central roles in setting the nation's health policy agenda, as they do subsequently in the development of legislation and in the implementation and modification of policies. Whether such groups play their roles proactively by seeking to stimulate new policies that serve the interests of their members or reactively by seeking to block policy changes that they do not believe serve their members' best interests, they are an innate part of the public policymaking process. Interest groups provide their members a way to link their policy preferences into more powerful, collective voices that greatly increase the likelihood of significant influence on the public policymaking process. As well, these links can provide additional sources of information about strategically important issues in the public policy environments of healthcare organizations.

In a pluralistic political marketplace, even one influenced by certain members of the power elite to a degree disproportionate to their numbers, strategymakers of healthcare organizations have no real choice about whether to join interest groups. The relevant question about membership and participation is which group or groups to join. The choices are manifold.

Categories of Interest Groups

All strategymakers in healthcare organizations have ready access to membership in a wide variety of interest groups and to the collective influence such memberships afford. As was noted in the previous chapter, strategymakers in hospitals, for example, can join the AHA and their state hospital associations. If they prefer a collective voice that is more specifically focused on their policy interests, strategymakers in teaching hospitals can link their organizations to the COTH, those in children's hospitals can join the National Association of Children's Hospitals and Related Institutions, and those in investor-owned hospitals can align themselves with the FAHS. These choices represent only a sampling of possible relevant interest groups for strategymakers. Indeed, strategymakers in all healthcare organizations face a dizzying array of interest groups to consider. Table 6.1 suggests the breadth of choices, restricted to groups with a national membership, by category of interest groups.

There are also other ways to categorize interest groups. Kingdon (1995) categorizes the different types of interest groups as business and industry, professional, labor, public interest, and governmental officials acting as lobbyists. In his view, the lobbying of one level of government by officials of another level is akin to the activities of a public interest group.

Buchholz (1994) categorizes groups according to their primary purpose. In his approach, economic interest groups are those that are formed primarily to promote the economic self-interest of members. The AHA and the AMA, along with many other healthcare groups, are included in this category by Buchholz.

Solidarity groups, in his classification scheme, are groups that are based at least in part on feelings of common identity based on a shared characteristic such as race, sex, or age. Examples include the National Association for the Advancement of Colored People (NAACP) and the National Organization for Women (NOW), and specifically in healthcare such organizations as the Women and Health Roundtable and the American Medical Women's Association.

The third category in Buchholz's scheme contains the public interest groups. In his view, these groups "do not necessarily appeal to the economic self-interest of their members, nor do they share common characteristics such as a solidarity group, but exist to promote noneconomic interests such as the environment or equal opportunity" (Buchholz 1989,

Table 6.1   Categories of Healthcare Interest Groups

....

- **Health and medical groups,** such as American Hospital Association, American Association of Certified Orthoptists, and Association for Health Services Research;

- **Trade, business, and commercial groups,** such as Contact Lens Manufacturers Association, National Association of Medical Equipment Suppliers, and Public Relations Society of America;

- **Environmental groups,** such as Hazardous Materials Control Research Institute;

- **Legal, governmental, public administration, and military groups,** such as Association of Food and Drug Officials, American Academy of Forensic Psychology, and National Health Law Program;

- **Engineering, technological, and natural and social sciences groups,** such as Association of Cytogenetic Technologists, IEEE Engineering in Medicine and Biology Society, and National Society of Biomedical Equipment Technicians;

- **Educational groups,** such as American Association of Dental Schools, Council for Medical Affairs, and Association of Professors of Medicine;

- **Cultural groups,** such as Interagency Council on Library Resources for Nursing, Medical Library Association, and Hospital Audiences;

- **Social welfare groups,** such as National Association of Public Child Welfare Administrators, National Committee for Prevention of Child Abuse, and National Organization of Adolescent Pregnancy and Parenting;

- **Public affairs groups,** such as Council for Responsible Genetics, National Council Against Health Fraud, National Health Policy Forum, and Intergovernmental Health Policy Project;

- **Religious groups,** such as American Baptist Homes and Hospitals Association, American Association of Pastoral Counselors, and Association for Clinical Pastoral Education;

- **Athletic and sports groups,** such as American Medical Athletic Association, North American Society for the Psychology of Sport and Physical Activity, and American Fitness Association; and

- **Labor unions, associations, and federations,** such as National Federation of Housestaff Organizations and Federation of Nurses and Health Professionals.

....

Source: *Lexikon* (p. xii) 1994 by M. R. O'Leary. Adapted by permission of Joint Commission on Accreditation of Healthcare Organizations.

139). Public interest groups are organizations that seek "a collective good, the achievement of which will not selectively and materially benefit the membership or activists of the organization" (Berry 1977, 7). Common Cause, which advocates openness and fairness in government, is an example of a public interest group. Other such groups seek to speak for those who cannot speak for themselves, such as children, animals, and the mentally ill. Some, such as the Sierra Club and the Audubon Society, pursue an environmentalist agenda on behalf of the public.

A third approach to categorizing interest groups is used by Lineberry, Edwards, and Wattenberg (1995) to cluster groups into those that address mainly economic issues, others that concern themselves with issues of energy and the environment, and still others that focus on equality issues. In this approach, equality interest groups are quite similar to the solidarity groups described by Buchholz. Although the Fourteenth Amendment to the U.S. Constitution guarantees equal protection under the law, American history clearly shows how difficult this equality has been to achieve. Interest groups such as the NAACP and NOW have made equality at the polls, in the workplace, in education, in housing, and in other facets of American life their central public policy goal (Kluger 1976; McGlen and O'Connor 1983).

Environmental groups, in their dedication to promoting pollution control and wilderness protection, have exerted significant influence on the public policymaking process, especially since the early 1970s. Their highly visible opposition to strip mining, the Alaskan oil pipeline, offshore oil drilling, and the construction and operation of nuclear power plants, for example, have brought the environmental groups into direct conflict with the nation's energy producers. The frequent and fervent conflicts between the environmental and energy interests in the United States have made the groups representing these interests prominent enough in the nation's public policymaking in the past two decades to earn them a category of their own in the view of many observers.

By far the largest category of interest groups in the Lineberry, Edwards, and Wattenberg approach, as in the one developed by Buchholz and indeed as in all categorizations of interest groups, are those in which the economic interests of members are the primary focus. All interest groups prefer public policies that favor their members; even the public interest groups seek to achieve their members' aims even though there may be no direct tangible benefits for the members as individuals. Economic advantages, however, are direct, tangible, and very important to a great many interest groups. Feldstein (1988) notes, for example, that healthcare provider interest groups seek through influencing the public policymaking process to accomplish such purposes as increasing the demand for members' services, limiting competitors, permitting members to charge the highest possible prices for their services, and lowering their members' operating costs as much as possible. Similarly, interest groups representing business interests or consumers seek through public policies to minimize the costs of these services to their members.

Among the categories of interest groups, those organized to serve the economic interests of their members are by wide margins the ones most likely to attract strategymakers in healthcare organizations, at least in terms of their strategymaking responsibilities. No matter what the basis for their formation or for their attractiveness to strategymakers, however, it is the functions performed by interest groups that lie at the heart of their appeal. These functions are examined in the next section.

Functions of Interest Groups

In addition to thinking about interest groups according to different categories, it is useful to consider them in terms of the functions they perform for their members. Although the primary function of many groups is to serve the economic self-interest of their members, groups also perform other functions of significant value to their members (Ornstein and Elder 1978).

Symbolic and Ideological Functions

Some interest groups perform valuable symbolic functions for their members, and in doing so, such groups provide their members with opportunities to express some of the personal interests or values they hold. In fact, the simple expressive action of joining a particular interest group can serve to clarify or reinforce one's professional identity or to provide legitimacy for certain ideas or values held to be important by the person who holds them. Many strategymakers in healthcare organizations, for example, join the ACHE in part because taking this action helps them to identify and define themselves professionally. Other professional associations or societies such as the American Bar Association, AMA, or American Political Science Association serve similar symbolic functions for their members because membership emphasizes their professional identities as lawyers, physicians, or political scientists.

Closely related to their symbolic functions, some groups serve ideological functions for their members. An interest group can provide an outlet for the ideological interests of its members, whether in some specific aspect of American life, such as abortion rights or environmental conservation, or in broader movements, such as political conservatism or liberalism. Symbolic and ideological functions are essentially psychological in nature and stand in contrast to certain more concrete functions.

Concrete Functions

Ornstein and Elder (1978) consider the concrete functions of interest groups to include such things as assisting their members to pursue economic goals or being instrumental in the achievement of other noneconomic goals that the members might have. When an interest group advances the economic interests of its individual or organizational members, it is performing a very concrete function for them. In addition to advancing the economic interests of its members, interest groups pursue other very concrete functions related to what are essentially noneconomic goals of their members. Such goals can nevertheless be among the important strategic goals of members.

In the healthcare domain, interest groups whose members have strategic goals that include changing health-related behaviors in areas such as sexual practices, smoking habits, or alcohol and drug use can be instrumental in helping the groups' members achieve these goals. Instrumental assistance is made in the same form in these cases as that used in pursuing economic benefits for interest group members; that is, an interest group's instrumentality in both cases is through influencing public policies that support desired outcomes. In one case, the desired outcome may be to increase the incomes of members. In the other case, the outcome sought may be to increase funding streams to support education or other prevention efforts to change human behavior.

A Cross-Cutting Function: The Provision of Information

The provision of useful information to their members, and to policymakers and the public on behalf of their members, is a very important function performed by interest groups. The information function is useful to members in support of both their analysis and influencing responsibilities regarding public policy environments. The information function cuts across the other functions that interest groups perform. Information supports the successful performance of the symbolic and ideological functions as well as of the more concrete economic and noneconomic instrumentality functions. Information can enhance the performance of these other functions and improve the likelihood that the purposes to which they are directed can be achieved.

The information function is a key mechanism of interest groups' influence with policymakers and, through them, of their influence in the policymaking process. Although the information supplied by interest groups tends to emphasize and support the policy preferences of the groups' members, it can nevertheless be useful to policymakers. The primary requisite for the information's usefulness is its accuracy. Interest groups do not benefit from nor do they want reputations for being careless or intentionally misleading with the information they supply to policymakers. Few things impair their effectiveness more quickly or seriously.

Information is provided to policymakers by interest groups in three different ways. The most direct route is through conversation or correspondence with policymakers. A semidirect route is through conversation or correspondence with the staffs of policymakers. A third, indirect, route is through supplying information to the media or through advertisements designed to influence the public's position on an issue and, through this, to influence policymakers.

The first two approaches—direct and semidirect means of providing information to policymakers—require, above all else, access to policymakers and to their staffs. Access to policymakers and the quality of the access—number of points of access, the ability to access key policymakers, and the warmth of the policymakers' reception—are among the most valuable assets any interest group can possess (Ornstein and Elder 1978; Wolfinger, Shapiro, and Greenstein 1980).

Interest groups also routinely supply information to their members about aspects of the public policy environment that are of importance to the members. As with an interest group's effectiveness in providing information to policymakers, access is also crucial to the way they are able to provide useful information gleaned from the public policy environment to their members. Information based on announced decisions and "done deals" is not nearly as valuable as information that accurately reflects policy decisions in the making, especially when there might still be time to adequately prepare for their effect or to influence them.

As important as interest groups can be as sources of information about the public policy environments of healthcare organizations, however, strategymakers are often more interested in how much assistance groups can provide to them in their efforts at influencing the policymaking process to the strategic advantage of their organizations.

How Interest Groups Influence Public Policymaking

Interest groups rely heavily on four tactics as their means of influencing the public policymaking process: lobbying, electioneering, litigation, and, especially more recently, influencing public opinion in order that it might in turn influence the policymaking process to the groups' advantage (Lineberry, Edwards, and Wattenberg 1995; Kingdon 1995). Each of these tactics is described in turn in the following sections.

Lobbying

Lobbying is a widespread influencing tactic, one with very deep roots in American public policymaking. "Lobbying is as old as legislation and pressure groups are as old as politics" (Schriftgeisser 1951, 3). Although lobbying conjures in the minds of many people a negative image of money exchanging hands for political favors and back room deals, lobbying is essentially nothing more than communicating with public policymakers for the purpose of influencing their decisions to be more favorable to, or at least consistent with, the preferences of those doing the lobbying (Buchholz 1994; Milbrath 1963).

The words lobbying and lobbyists arose in reference to the place where such activities first took place. In early Washington, D.C., before members of Congress had either offices or telephones, certain people who sought to influence their thinking waited for them and talked to them in the lobbies of buildings the members of Congress frequented. The original practitioners of this influencing tactic spent so much time in lobbies that they came, naturally enough, to be called lobbyists, and their work termed lobbying.

Like many other groups of people, lobbyists come in great variety. The vast majority of them operate in an ethical and professional manner, effectively representing the legitimate interests of the groups they serve. The few, however, who behave in heavy-handed, even illegal ways have in certain ways smudged the reputations of all those who do this work. Their image is further affected by the fact that their work, if it is properly done, is essentially selfish in nature. Lobbyists seek to persuade others that their position, which is really the position of the interests that they represent, is the correct one. Their whole professional purpose is to persuade others to make decisions that are in the best interests of those who employ or retain the lobbyists.

Studies as well as opinions on the effectiveness of the lobbying tactic as a means of influencing the public policymaking process are mixed at best (Bauer, Pool, and Dexter 1963; Milbrath 1963; Kingdon 1995). There is no doubt that lobbying has an impact on the policymaking process, but it seems to work best when applied to policymakers who are already committed to, or who are at least sympathetic to, the lobbyist's position on a public policy issue (Lineberry, Edwards, and Wattenberg, 1995). Lobbyists certainly played a prominent role in the defeat of President Clinton's 1993 Health Security Act bill. Similarly, they played a significant role in the repeal of the 1988 Catastrophic Health Care Act. In part, the ambivalence over the role of lobbying in influencing policymaking derives from the difficulty inherent in isolating its effect from some of the other tactics discussed below.

Whatever degree of influence lobbyists do exert on the public policymaking process is made possible by several well-understood sources of their influence with policymakers. Ornstein and Elder (1978) identify five ways that lobbyists can be of direct help to a member of Congress, each of which can be extended to other policymakers.

- Lobbyists are an important source of information for policymakers. Although most policymakers must be concerned with many policy issues simultaneously, most lobbyists can focus and specialize. They can become quite expert, and can draw on the insight of other experts, in the areas they represent.

- Lobbyists can help policymakers with the development and execution of political strategy. Lobbyists typically are politically savvy and can provide "free consulting" to policymakers they choose to assist.

- Lobbyists can assist policymakers, at least those who are elected, in their reelection efforts. (More about electioneering is said in the next section.) This assistance can take several forms, including campaign contributions, votes, and workers for campaigns.

- Lobbyists can be important sources of innovative ideas for policy-makers, who are judged on the quality of their ideas as well as on their abilities to have their ideas translated into effective policies. For most policymakers, few gifts are as valued as a really good idea. This is especially so when policymakers can turn ideas into bills that bear their names.

- Finally, lobbyists can be friends with policymakers. Lobbyists often are gregarious and interesting people in their own rights. They entertain, sometimes lavishly, and they are socially engaging. Many of them have social and educational backgrounds that are similar to those of policymakers. In fact, many lobbyists have been policymakers earlier in their careers. It is neither unusual nor surprising for lobbyists and policymakers to become friends.

Electioneering

The effective use of the electioneering tactic for influencing the policy-making process is based on the simple notion that policymakers who are sympathetic to a group's interests are far more likely to be influenced in their policymaking by the group's policy preferences than are policy-makers who are not sympathetic. Thus, interest groups seek to elect and keep in office policymakers who they view as sympathetic to the interests of the group's members. Electioneering, or using the resources at their disposal to aid candidates for political office, is a common means through which interest groups seek to exert their influence on the policymaking process. Many groups have considerable resources to devote to this tactic.

Interest groups, to varying degrees, have a family of resources that involve electoral advantages or disadvantages for political candidates. "Some groups—because of their geographical dispersion in congressional districts throughout the country; their ability to mobilize their members and sympathizers; and their numbers, status, or wealth—are thought to have an ability to affect election outcomes" (Kingdon 1995, 51).

One of the most visible aspects of the electioneering tactic is the channeling of money into the campaign finances of their supporters and sympathizers through political action committees or PACs. This source of funds now covers nearly half the costs of congressional elections in the United States (Lineberry, Edwards, and Wattenberg 1995). As Table 6.2 illustrates, healthcare interest groups participate heavily in this form of electioneering.

PACs are indeed important sources of influence for interest groups. However, the most influential groups tend to have multiple ways of exerting their influence through lobbying and electioneering activities. The hospital industry is a notable example. The AHA is a leading campaign contributor through its PAC. In addition, however, it has many other resources at its disposal. As Kingdon (1995) has pointed out, every congressional district has hospitals whose trustees are community leaders and whose managers and physicians are typically articulate and respected in their communities. These spokespersons can be mobilized to support sympathetic candidates or to contact their representatives directly regarding any policy decision.

Referring to the Carter administration's proposed Hospital Cost Containment Act of 1977 (Hughes et al. 1978), one policymaker challenged the wisdom of the administration's decision to take on this influential group with the following words:

> The whole cost containment thing is a quagmire. I don't know how in the hell the administration got involved with it as their first move [in the healthcare domain]. Here you have thousands of hospitals in this country. More than half of them are community hospitals, and you know what that means. There's a lot of community pride wrapped up in them; they've been financed by bake sales. "It's *our* hospital." Others of them are proprietary hospitals, owned by politically powerful physicians. The rest of them have some religious affiliation and here they are doing the Lord's work. Why would you want to take them on? Dumb, dumb, dumb. (Kingdon 1995, 51–52)

Table 6.2   Healthcare Industry Political Action Committee (PAC) Contributions to Congressional Candidates and Soft Money Contributions to National Political Party Committees, July 1985–June 1995

Health Insurance Companies	$ 25.5 million
Physicians	23.1 million
Hospitals and Nursing Homes	9.7 million

Source: Common Cause News Release, December 1, 1995.

As Ornstein and Elder observe, "The ability of a group to mobilize its membership strength for political action is a highly valuable resource; a small group that is politically active and cohesive can have more political impact than a large, politically apathetic, and unorganized group" (1978, 74). The ability to mobilize people and other resources at the grassroots level helps explain the relative capabilities of various groups to influence policymakers and, through them, the policymaking process. Table 6.3 ranks the more influential healthcare interest groups according to the opinions of congressional staff who were surveyed. The groups at the top of the list have particularly strong grassroots organizations to call into play in the exercise of their lobbying and electioneering tactics.

Litigation

A third common tactic available to interest groups in their efforts to influence the policymaking process is litigation. As was discussed in Chapter 5, interest groups, acting on behalf of their members, seek to influence policymaking through litigation in which they challenge existing policies, seek to stimulate new policies, or try to alter certain aspects of the implementation of policies. Use of the litigation tactic, in both state and federal courts, is a widespread and increasingly used tactic in the efforts of interest groups to influence policymaking in the healthcare domain.

Table 6.3 Influential Healthcare Interest Groups

1. Hospice Association of America
2. American Hospital Association
3. American Medical Association
4. Group Health Association of America
5. National Association for Home Care
6. Health Insurance Association of America
7. American Health Care Association
8. American Dental Association
9. National Association of Social Workers
10. American Nurses Association
11. American Federation of Home Health Agencies
12. American Association for Homes and Services for the Aging
13. National Association of Medical Equipment Suppliers

Source: American Hospital Association. "AHA Receives High Marks on the Hill." *AHA News* 31 (24), June 12, 1995, 3; reprinted with permission from American Hospital Publishing, Inc. Data reflect average scores in a survey of congressional staff conducted for the National Association for Home Care by Fleishman-Hillard Inc.

Several examples of the use of the courts in influencing policymaking were described in Chapter 5. In one of the cases cited there, a group of commercial insurers and HMOs and New York City challenged the state of New York's practice of adding a surcharge to certain hospital bills to raise money to fund healthcare for indigent people (Green 1995). This case was heard by the U.S. Supreme Court. Because its outcome was of considerable importance to their members, a number of healthcare interest groups filed *amicus curiae* briefs as a means of influencing the court's decision. Through such written depositions, groups state their collective positions on issues and describe how the decision in the case will affect their members. This practice is widely used by healthcare interest groups as well as by groups in other domains. Through the practice, the Supreme Court has been accessible to these groups who, in expressing their views, have helped determine which cases the court will hear as well as how they rule in them (Caldeira and Wright 1990). This practice is also frequently and effectively used by interest groups in lower courts as well.

One particularly effective use of the litigation tactic is to turn to the courts to help fill in the specific details of how vague pieces of legislation will actually be implemented. This practice provides opportunities for interest groups to exert enormous influence on policymaking overall by influencing the rules and administrative practices that guide the implementation of public statutes or laws. Recall from the discussion of this point in Chapter 3 that the implementation rules and administrative decisions made by implementing organizations are themselves authoritative decisions that fit the definition of public policies.

Shaping Public Opinion

Knowing that policymakers are influenced by the opinions held by the electorate, many interest groups employ the tactic of seeking to shape public opinion as another means through which they might ultimately influence the policymaking process. This tactic, for example, was used extensively in the congressional debate over national healthcare reform in 1993 and 1994. It is estimated that interest groups spent more than $50 million seeking to shape public opinion on the issues involved in the debate. For example, anyone who followed the debate even peripherally became familiar with the health insurance industry's "Harry and Louise" ads.[1] The extensive healthcare reform debate of the early 1990s

---

1. Harry and Louise were the names given to the actors in a series of television ads that were sponsored by the Health Insurance Association of America as part of its campaign to shape public opinion about healthcare reform, especially the Clinton plan for reform. As described by Johnson and Broder (1996, 16), this advertising campaign "featured Mr. and Mrs. Average American Couple,

was not the first use of the shaping of public opinion tactic by healthcare interest groups, however.

The congressional debate over the Medicare legislation in the 1960s was fueled by intense opposition to the legislation in some quarters, especially by the AMA. The American public had rarely if ever experienced so feverish a campaign to shape opinions as it was exposed to in the period leading up to enactment of the Medicare legislation in 1965. Among the many activities undertaken in the campaign to influence public opinion, (and through this, policymakers) perhaps none is more entertaining in hindsight and certainly few are more representative of the campaign's tone and intensity as one action taken by the AMA. As part of its campaign to influence public opinion on this matter, the AMA sent every physician's spouse a recording, with the advice that they should play the record for their friends and neighbors. The idea was to encourage these people to write letters in opposition to the legislation to their representatives in Congress. Near the end of the recording, these words are heard:

> Write those letters now; call your friends and tell them to write them. If you don't, this program, I promise you, will pass just as surely as the sun will come up tomorrow. And behind it will come other federal programs that will invade every area of freedom as we have known it in this country. Until one day . . . we will awake to find that we have socialism. And if you don't do this, and I don't do it, one of these days you and I are going to spend our sunset years telling our children and our children's children what it was like in America when men were free. (Skidmore 1970, 138)

The words are made all the more interesting by the fact that the voice on the recording, easily recognizable three decades after the record was made, is that of Ronald Reagan.

There is no firm evidence of the effect of the appeals to public opinion made by interest groups on either policymakers or policymaking (Lineberry, Edwards, and Wattenberg 1995). The extent and persistence of the practice, nevertheless, suggests that interest groups believe that it does make a difference. One variable does clearly mitigate the usefulness of the tactic and makes its use by interest groups vastly more difficult: the heterogeneity of the American population.

A great myth about democracies is that their voters reach consensus, and when a consensus is not possible then at least a majority viewpoint

---

'Harry and Louise,' expressing fears that the Clinton plan would restrict their freedom to choose and result in 'government-run health care.' 'There has to be a better way,' Louise says to Harry, in a punch line that was beginning to become familiar to Americans assessing how the Clinton reform would affect them."

emerges to guide policymakers in their decisions. Sometimes this happens, but rarely on issues as complex as those typically arising in the healthcare domain. For example, in the debate over healthcare reform in 1994 there was a majority viewpoint that healthcare reform was needed at the beginning of the debate. However, at no time during the debate was a public consensus achieved on the nature of the reform that should be undertaken. No feasible alternative for reform ever received majority support in any public opinion poll. During most of the debate, in fact, public opinion was approximately evenly divided among three possible reform options (Brodie and Blendon 1995).

Further complicating the potential usefulness of efforts by interest groups seeking to influence public opinion is the fact that on complex issues public opinion undergoes a series of evolutionary changes. Yankelovich (1992) has pointed out that the public's thinking on possible policy solutions to difficult problems evolves through predictable stages. These stages, as discussed in Chapter 3, begin with people becoming aware of a problem. Then, they begin an exploration, with varying degrees of success, of the problem and alternative solutions. Eventually, many of them reach judgments about the problem and how they think it should be addressed through policymaking. A consequence of this evolutionary thought process is that the heterogeneous mass of people who are the American public will likely be scattered all along the evolutionary continuum on complex issues.

Using lobbying, electioneering, litigation and their efforts to shape public opinion as tactics, interest groups influence the public policymaking process to the strategic advantage of their members. The degree of success they achieve in this is highly dependent on the resources at their disposal. The most important of these resources are considered in the next section.

The Resources of Interest Groups

Interest groups vary along many dimensions including membership, purposes, philosophies, and the resources at their disposal. Ornstein and Elder (1978) categorize the resources of interest groups into:

- physical resources, especially money and the number of members;
- organizational resources such as the quality of a group's leadership, the degree of unity or cohesion among its members, and the group's ability to mobilize its membership for political purposes;
- political resources such as expertise in the intricacies of the public policymaking process and political reputation for being able to influence the process ethically and effectively;

- motivational resources such as the strength of ideological conviction among the membership; and
- intangible resources such as the overall status or prestige of a group.

The particular mix of these resources available to an interest group, as well as how effectively the resources are used by the group, help determine the group's performance. A group's performance in assisting its members in the achievement of their strategic goals by influencing the public policymaking process is affected not only by the group's resources but also by how the group's resources compare to those of other groups that may be pursuing competing or conflicting outcomes from the policymaking process (Feldstein 1988; Kingdon 1995; Lineberry, Edwards, and Wattenberg 1995).

One particularly important group resource is the relative proportion of its potential members who have become actual members. Although it seems somewhat counterintuitive, small groups typically perform better than large groups in exerting influence on the policymaking process. Essentially, this phenomenon exists because small groups tend to have greater proportions of potential members who are actual members. "Part of a group's stock in trade in affecting all phases of policy making—agendas, decisions, or implementation—is its ability to convince government officials that it speaks with one voice and truly represents the preferences of its members" (Kingdon 1995, 52). Large numbers of potential members can, of course, work to a group's advantage. Converting many potential members into actual members might result in more financial resources or it might result in a group having members living in every congressional district, for example.

However, the costs of organizing a large group, especially if their interests are not extremely concordant and focused, can be quite high, higher perhaps than the benefits members might gain from membership. Smaller groups tend to be easier and less costly to organize than larger groups. Thus, the ratio of benefits-to-costs favors the formation and maintenance of small groups. It also means that smaller groups are more likely than larger ones to have greater proportions of potential members who actually join the group. When groups do not represent all of their potential members, they cannot speak with a common voice and are thus less influential in the policymaking arena as a consequence.

To gain the cohesive benefit of having a large proportion of potential members of a group actually join the group, what is called the free-rider problem must be overcome (Olson 1965). The larger the group, the more difficult it is to overcome this problem. All interest groups seek to provide collective goods for their members. In the process, when they succeed, they may also provide the benefits of the collective goods for others who are not members of the group. A collective good is something of value, the benefits of which cannot be withheld from a group's actual members or from its potential members. Better reimbursement rates for all hospitals under the Medicare program or more generous overall funding for AIDS research are collective goods that can benefit all hospitals or all AIDS researchers. It does not matter that some of the beneficiaries do not belong to the interest groups whose efforts secured the benefits.

Large interest groups can certainly be effective. Once they are organized, in fact, they can be extremely effective. However, it is much more difficult for them to organize in the first place. This frequently means that small, cohesive interest groups have an advantage over larger ones in the competition to influence public policymaking. They gain their advantage primarily because they are more likely to represent a greater proportion of potential members. It is easier for them to speak with one voice for their members than is the case for groups that only represent a small fraction of their potential members or who have memberships that are divided on policy issues.

Summary

James Madison's hope for a government in which interest groups are permitted to participate freely in seeking to influence policymaking on behalf of their members has come to a full realization as the nation approaches the twenty-first century. However, it is not quite so clear if his hope that many groups participating in the policymaking process would ensure than none of them gained too much influence has been realized. The pluralists argue that the participants in the large array of competing interest groups counterbalance each other in the political marketplace and that something akin to the public interest emerges from this competition. In contrast, those who take an elitist view argue that the power elite in society dominate public policymaking; they shape the formulation of policies and control the implementation of policies through their powerful roles in the nation's economic and social systems.

The conclusion reached is that neither the pluralist nor the elitist perspectives alone explain how the interests of individuals, acting through their interest groups, relate to the public policymaking process. Clearly, everyone's interests are affected by the process, although not to the same degree. In turn, many if not all interests can influence the policymaking process through participation in interest groups, although not everyone influences the process to an equal degree. Both approaches have something of value to contribute to strategymakers in healthcare organizations as they consider the roles that interest groups might play in their efforts to both discern and influence their public policy environments.

As a means of considering the various types of interest groups at work in the American political economy, several categories of groups are presented. It is noted that among the various categories of interest groups, those organized to serve the economic interests of their members are by far the ones most likely to appeal to strategymakers in healthcare organizations, at least in regard to their concerns about their strategy-making responsibilities.

The several functions performed by interest groups for their members are described. Although emphasis is placed on the concrete function of serving the economic interests of their members, the symbolic and ideological functions are also discussed. The provision of useful information to their members as well as the provision of information to others, such as policymakers and the public, on behalf of their members is discussed as a very important cross-cutting function that is performed by interest groups.

It is noted that interest groups rely on four principle tactics to influence the public policymaking process: lobbying, electioneering, litigation, and, more recently, seeking to influence public opinion in order that it might in turn influence the policymaking process to the groups' advantage. In using these tactics to influence the public policymaking process to the strategic advantage of their members, the degree of success these groups achieve is affected by the resources at their disposal.

The most important of these resources are discussed in the chapter and include physical resources, especially money; organizational resources such as the quality of a group's leadership and the degree of cohesion among its members; political resources such as expertise in the intricacies of the public policymaking process and political reputation for being able to influence the process ethically and effectively; motivational resources such as the strength of ideological conviction among the membership; and such intangible resources as a group's prestige. The chapter concludes with a discussion of a particularly important group resource: the relative proportion of its potential members who have decided to become actual members. There is an advantage for any interest group in being able to represent its potential members as a single voice.

References

American Hospital Association. 1995. "AHA Receives High Marks on the Hill." *AHA News* 31 (24): 3.

Bauer, R. A., I. de S. Pool, and L. A. Dexter. 1963. *American Business and Public Policy.* New York: Atherton.

Berry, J. M. 1977. *Lobbying for the People*. Princeton, NJ: Princeton University Press.

Bibfeldt, F. 1958. *Paradoxes Observed*. Chicago: Perspective Press.

Brodie, M., and R. J. Blendon. 1995. "The Public's Contribution to Congressional Gridlock on Health Care Reform." *Journal of Health Politics, Policy and Law* 20 (2): 403–10.

Buchholz, R. A. 1994. *Business Environment and Public Policy: Implications for Management,* 5th ed. Englewood Cliffs, NJ: Prentice Hall.

Caldeira, G. A., and J. R. Wright. 1990. "*Amici Curiae* Before the Supreme Court: Who Participates, When, and How Much?" *Journal of Politics* 52 (August): 782–804.

Common Cause News Release, December 1, 1995.

Dye, T. R. 1990. *Who's Running America? The Bush Era*, 5th ed. Englewood Cliffs, NJ: Prentice Hall.

———. 1995. *Understanding Public Policy*, 8th ed. Englewood Cliffs, NJ: Prentice Hall.

Dye, T. R., and H. Zeigler. 1975. *The Irony of Democracy*, 3rd ed. New York: Wadsworth Publishing Company, Inc.

Encyclopedia of Associations. 1993. Detroit, MI: Gale.

Feldstein, P. J. 1988. *The Politics of Health Legislation: An Economic Perspective*. Ann Arbor, MI: Health Administration Press.

Green, J. 1995. "High-Court Ruling Protects Hospital-bill Surcharges." *AHA News* 31 (18): 1.

Hughes, E. F. X., D. P. Baron, D. A. Dittman, B. S. Friedman, B. B. Longest, Jr., M. V. Pauly, and K. R. Smith. 1978. *Hospital Cost Containment Programs: A Policy Analysis*. Cambridge, MA: Ballinger Publishing Company.

Johnson, H., and D. S. Broder. 1996. *The System: The American Way of Politics at the Breaking Point*. Boston: Little, Brown and Company.

Kingdon, J. W. 1995. *Agendas, Alternatives, and Public Policies*, 2nd ed. New York: HarperCollins College Publishers.

Kluger, R. 1976. *Simple Justice*. New York: Knopf.

Leary, M. R. 1994. *Lexikon*. Oakbrook Terrace, IL: Joint Commission on Accreditation of Heathcare Organization.

Lineberry, R. L., G. C. Edwards, III, and M. P. Wattenberg. 1995. *Government in America*, 2nd ed. New York: HarperCollins College Publishers.

Lowi, T. J. 1979. *The End of Liberalism*, 2nd ed. New York: Norton.

Madison, J., A. Hamilton, and J. Jay. *The Federalist Papers*. New York: Modern Library, no date.

McGlen, N., and K. O'Connor. 1983. *Women's Rights: The Struggle for Equality in the Nineteenth and Twentieth Centuries*. New York: Praeger.

Milbrath, L. W. 1963. *The Washington Lobbyists*. Chicago: Rand McNally.

Moe, T. 1980. *The Organization of Interests*. Chicago: University of Chicago Press.

Morone, J. A. 1990. *The Democratic Wish: Popular Participation and the Limits of American Government*. New York: Basic Books.

Olson, M. 1965. *The Logic of Collective Action*. Cambridge, MA: Harvard University Press.

Ornstein, N. J., and S. Elder. 1978. *Interest Groups, Lobbying and Policymaking*. Washington, DC: Congressional Quarterly Press.

Peters, B. G. 1986. *American Public Policy: Promise and Performance*, 2nd ed. Chatham, NJ: Chatham House.

Scholzman, K. L., and J. T. Tierney. 1986. *Organized Interests and American Democracy*. New York: Harper & Row.

Schriftgeisser, K. 1951. *The Lobbyists*. Boston: Little, Brown and Company.

Skidmore, M. 1970. *Medicare and the American Rhetoric of Reconciliation*. Tuscaloosa, AL: University of Alabama Press.

Truman, D. 1971. *The Governmental Process*, 2nd ed. New York: Knopf.

Wilson, J. Q. 1973. *Political Organizations*. New York: Basic Books.

Wolfinger, R. E., M. Shapiro, and F. I. Greenstein. 1980. *Dynamics of American Politics*, 2nd ed. Englewood Cliffs, NJ: Prentice Hall.

Yankelovich, D. 1992. "How Public Opinion Really Works." *Fortune* (5 October): 102–8.

7

An Applied Example: Strategymaking at the University of Texas Health Center at Tyler

The concepts and techniques presented in the previous chapters are applied to an example that is drawn from the world of strategymaking practice. A brief history of the University of Texas Health Center at Tyler and a description of the situation facing its strategymakers is presented. The selection of the Health Center is based on its usefulness as an illustration of a complex strategymaking situation, not because of any particular decisions and actions of this organization's strategymakers.

Following the history are a series of questions about the strategymakers and their strategymaking. Answers to these questions are provided, with reference to the chapters in the book where related material is found. The case history is adapted by Mark J. Kroll and Beaufort B. Longest, Jr. from Dr. Kroll's long version of the case, "University of Texas Health Center at Tyler."

Today, the University of Texas Health Center at Tyler is a healthcare organization with a tripartite mission of patient care, medical education, and research. The center's complex mission has evolved considerably over its lifetime. The evolution of the center's mission as well as the strategymaking that has both guided and been influenced by this evolving mission illustrate many of the key elements that are of concern to those with strategic responsibilities in contemporary healthcare organizations.

The Center's History

The East Texas Tuberculosis Sanatorium, the organization that eventually became the University of Texas Health Center at Tyler, was founded in 1947 as a state tuberculosis sanatorium by act of the fiftieth Texas Legislature. The state of Texas established the organization on the site of a deactivated World War II army infantry training base located just outside Tyler, in the region known as East Texas. The state acquired 614 acres of land along with the buildings that had served as the base hospital from the federal government. Most of the base's 1,000 beds were in rows of wooden barracks, with each barrack accommodating 25 beds in an open ward. Patients were first admitted to the sanatorium in 1949. Since its establishment, the organization has changed dramatically in a number of ways. Its structure and operations have been adapted to an evolving mission and to the changing healthcare needs of the citizens of Texas, especially those of the East Texas region.

In 1951, the Texas Legislature changed the center's name to the East Texas Tuberculosis Hospital. This new name, in which the word *hospital* replaced *sanatorium*, reflected a change in the center's mission from simple custodial care to an emphasis on treatment using newly developed drugs.

Although several legislative acts passed during the 1950s changed the organization's governing authority, it was not until 1969 that its mission was extended beyond the care and treatment of patients with tuberculosis. In that year, the Texas Legislature authorized the organization to develop pilot programs aimed at treating other respiratory diseases, such as asthma, lung cancer, chronic bronchitis, emphysema, and occupational diseases related to asbestos exposure. In 1971, the legislature gave the organization a still broader mission by incorporating education and research into the existing patient care mission. At that time, the organization's name was changed to the East Texas Chest Hospital.

In 1977, a state senator from Tyler sponsored legislation that transferred control of the hospital to the Board of Regents of the University of Texas System. This legislation authorized the regents to operate the institution as a teaching hospital—a unit of the University of Texas System—and to change its name to the University of Texas Health Center at Tyler. It also reaffirmed the organization's mission as serving as a primary state referral center for patient care, operating education programs, and conducting research on the diseases of the chest.

As its mission has evolved, the Health Center's organizational structure, operations, and physical configuration have also changed. In 1957, for example, the state completed a 320-bed, six-story brick and masonry structure that replaced the original wooden barracks. An outpatient clinic was added to the hospital in 1970. In 1976, the state appropriated money for construction of a replacement hospital facility. Today, the Health Center operates 166 beds, recording about 3,400 inpatient admissions annually.

The Watson W. Wise Medical Research Library was completed and dedicated in 1984. This facility supported the work of a growing research faculty and the addition of new departments such as biochemistry, microbiology, and physiology. The research library has been instrumental in establishing the East Texas Sciences Library Consortium, which includes other hospitals and colleges in the area. This consortium serves as a valuable resource for medical professionals in the entire East Texas region.

In 1987, the Health Center's Biomedical Research Building was completed. This was followed in 1991 with the groundbreaking for a $12.5 million expansion of the Health Center's ambulatory care facilities. Completed in early 1996, the ambulatory care center can accommodate more than 120,000 outpatient encounters annually. Outpatient services available at the Health Center now include family practice, breast diagnostics, sleep evaluation, occupational medicine, oncology, general internal medicine, urgent care, adult asthma, opthamology, travel medicine, sports medicine, orthopedics, same day surgery, gastroenterology services, rheumatology, cardiology, and pediatric pulmonary, allergy, and immunology.

Reflecting the pattern of expanding programs at the Health Center, surgeons began to perform open heart surgery there in 1983, the same year in which the Health Center was designated as one of the state's regional cystic fibrosis centers. In 1985, it was designated as a national cystic fibrosis satellite center. Another important programmatic development took place in the early 1990s. The Health Center established the Texas Institute of Occupational Safety and Health, which assists area companies and their employees by providing preventive medicine programs, physical examinations, and the monitoring of environmental health hazards in the workplace.

In 1985 in cooperation with two other Tyler hospitals the first postgraduate medical education program in East Texas, residency training in family practice, was inaugurated at the center. Today the Health Center operates an active three-year postgraduate residency program in family practice, the only one of its kind in East Texas. About 65 percent of its graduates are placed in East Texas communities, many of which have no other primary care physicians.

Grant research funding has increased steadily at the Health Center. In 1983, funding was about $80,000 annually. Today, center scientists annually receive about $3 million in competitive grants from external sources such as the NIH, the Texas Affiliate of the American Heart Association, the American Lung Association of Texas, the Muscular Dystrophy Foundation, private foundations, and several industrial and pharmaceutical firms. Completion of the Biomedical Research Building in 1987, along with the recruitment of several new research scientists, has helped the Health Center aggressively pursue the research component of its mission.

Currently, the Health Center ranks eighth in Texas and first in the East Texas region in the amount of research being conducted, and leads the area in attracting biotechnology industries to the region. It was granted its first two biomedical research patents in fiscal year 1992, added two more in fiscal year 1993, and another is pending.

In 1993, the Health Center was granted $1 million over the biennium by the Texas Legislature to establish and operate the Center for Pulmonary Infectious Disease Control. This center is a locus for research, the development of medical protocols, and the dissemination of information regarding diseases of the lungs, particularly tuberculosis and drug-resistant tuberculosis. It makes the Health Center the leader in the battle against the resurgence of an old killer, tuberculosis, in Texas.

From its roots as a custodial care facility, the Health Center has evolved into a complex teaching hospital with a three-part mission of patient care, education, and research. In addition, the Health Center is the largest state employer in East Texas with more than 1,300 employees and an annual operating budget of approximately $65 million. The center also provides charity care, in the amount of more than $12 million annually, for Texans who need it.

The Center's Market

The Health Center is located in the middle of Smith County in East Texas. Two private hospitals share the Health Center's service area. These hospitals average between 12,000 and 16,000 inpatient admissions annually; each has an operating budget of approximately $100 million and a medical staff of about 300 physicians.

Many hospitals and physicians statewide refer patients to the Health Center for diagnosis and treatment, especially when pulmonary problems are suspected. In fact, the center typically draws patients from over half of the state's 254 counties. However, its primary service area is considered to be the 24 surrounding counties; the bulk of its patients come from this surrounding East Texas area. The center's strategymakers base their forecasts for future patient demand primarily on the demographics of this area, which, like the rest of the state, is increasing in population.

The population in the center's service area is expected to increase during the 1990s from 1,060,030 to as much as 1,295,949. Also, as elsewhere in Texas, the East Texas population that is 65 and older is expected to continue to increase dramatically.

Its patient base is vitally important to the center because its operating budget comprises general revenue appropriations from the state, research grant funding, and revenues from services provided to paying patients. Research grant funding has leveled off, and the state's general revenue appropriations have not kept pace with increasing expenses at the Health Center. This has put increased pressure on the Health Center to generate funds through its paying patient base. Related to this, although the Health Center continues its long-standing commitment to providing charity care, it has been forced to control these costs. For example, the center has been forced to limit the prescription drugs it provides free of charge to indigent patients and to restrict the amount of charity care provided in some of its clinics.

The Center's Regulatory Environment

Regulation is an integral part of the entire healthcare industry's macroenvironment; the Health Center is certainly no exception to this condition. Regulations that directly affect the center are promulgated by numerous government and industry agencies, including the HCFA, the DHHS, the FDA, the Texas Department of Health, and the Joint Commission on Accreditation of Healthcare Organizations (JCAHO). In addition, reflecting its ownership, operational regulations are imposed on the Health Center by the state of Texas and by the University of Texas System.

Like most healthcare organizations in the past decade, regulations associated with the prospective payment system for Medicare reimbursement for patient care have had significant impact on the Health Center. Currently, half of its patients are covered by Medicare. Under the provisions of the prospective payment system, hospitals are paid for treating Medicare patients on the basis of diagnosis-specific rates rather than on the basis of their actual costs, as was the case until these regulations were implemented in 1984.

The prognosis for future cuts in the Medicare program's reimbursement levels and in those of the state's Medicaid program is very serious for the Health Center. Not only would patient care revenues be affected, but the center's ability to recover some of the costs of its medical education programs, especially its family practice residency, is also threatened by changes in these programs.

The Center's Governance and Management

The University of Texas System is presided over by a board of regents whose members include business leaders, educators, and physicians and other professionals. Individually and collectively, the board's members have significant influence with the Texas Legislature through which they can secure funding for the university system and help shape legislation that is relevant to the system.

The board of regents sets the financial and operating guidelines of the University of Texas System through operating budgets, capital expenditure approvals, and program authorizations. The board essentially supports or rejects recommendations from the administrators of the universities and health centers in the system, including the center at Tyler. The board of regents implements its decisions through the chancellor of the University of Texas System.

The Health Center's top management is organized along functional lines according to business, research, educational, and patient care activities. The organization chart for the Health Center is illustrated in Figure 7.1.

The patient care, research, and medical education divisions are directed by the executive associate director, who is a physician as well as a research scientist. The incumbent is highly regarded for his skills as an administrator, physician, and researcher. This senior-level manager is supported by assistant administrators along functional lines: chief of staff and associate directors for patient services, for research, and for medical education. The business division of the center is directed by the executive associate director for administration and business affairs. This senior-level manager is supported by the associate director for fiscal affairs and by two other assistant directors.

The Center's Future

From a rather simple beginning, the Health Center has evolved into a complex organization. Its strategymakers now pursue a complex three-fold mission to provide patient care, to conduct research, and to provide education.

The center's patient care services currently include inpatient and ambulatory care services that are provided by a nationally recruited clinical staff. They provide a full range of services for cardiovascular diagnosis, treatment, and rehabilitation, including coronary angioplasty. Nationally known for its pulmonary disease capabilities, the Health Center has the most highly developed program for comprehensive evaluation and treatment of occupational lung diseases in Texas. Similarly, significant progress has been made in its research and education programs. However, the Health Center faces some difficult challenges and threats.

Changing economic conditions, recent and probably continuing reductions in both state and federal funding, and the increasing costs of fulfilling each part of its mission present substantial threats to which the Health Center's strategymakers must make strategic responses. Increasingly, the center's strategymakers, like those in other healthcare organizations across the nation, are challenged to analyze the center's public policy environment effectively and to influence this environment to the center's strategic advantage. The degree of success they achieve in fulfilling these responsibilities will heavily influence the future of the center.

Questions and Discussion

1. *Who are the strategymakers at the University of Texas Health Center at Tyler?*

As is discussed in Chapter 1, the strategymakers in any organization, alliance, or system of organizations, are its senior-level managers and those who sit on its governing board. As is further discussed in Chapter 4, senior-level managers occupy positions at or near the top of their organization and are responsible for its overall performance and condition. Their core work is to set the strategic direction of their organization. This strategic responsibility encompasses the diverse activities and efforts needed to establish suitable organizational objectives and to develop and implement the means of accomplishing them. When managers play strategic roles they must think about how to adapt their organizational domains to the external challenges and opportunities presented to them by their environments, including public policies.

At the University of Texas Health Center at Tyler, the strategymakers can be seen in Figure 7.1. They include the board of regents whose members set the financial and operational guidelines under which all units of the University of Texas System operate. The board implements its decisions through the chancellor of the University of Texas System. Thus, the chancellor is part of the strategic apex of the Health Center. Within the center, the director (the center's chief executive officer) along with the executive associate director in charge of research and education activities and the executive associate director for administration and business affairs form the senior management strategymaking group.

It is important to remember, as is discussed in Chapter 5, that the challenges of effective strategymaking are so great that the strategymakers in healthcare organizations typically cannot hope to meet these challenges successfully by relying exclusively on themselves and the use of their own internal organizational resources. Instead, in view of the dynamic set of forces and actors at work in their organization's public policy environment, strategymakers frequently seek the assistance of outside resources. The primary source of such assistance is the interest groups to which strategymakers and their organizations belong. This aspect of

Figure 7.1 Organization Chart: The University of Texas Health Center at Tyler

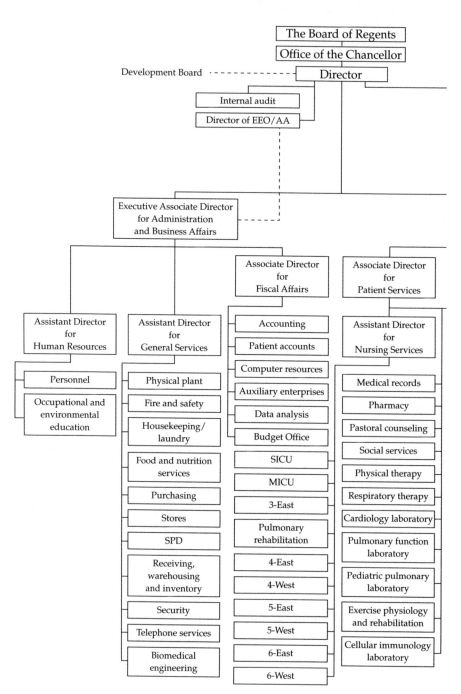

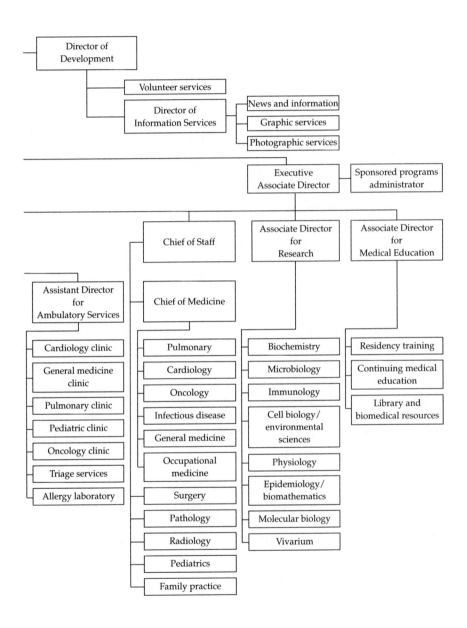

the efforts of strategymakers to succeed at analyzing and influencing the public policy environments of their organizations is covered in Chapter 6. The Health Center can turn for outside assistance to organizations such as the AHA and the COTH, for example.

2. *What responsibilities do the strategymakers at the Health Center have regarding its public policy environment?*
    The Health Center's external environment includes many variables that can influence strategymaking for it and ultimately its organizational performance. In addition to public policies, the Health Center, like all healthcare organizations, is affected by biological, cultural, demographic, ecological, economic, ethical, legal, psychological, social, and technological variables. Although all of these environmental variables affect the center, this book concentrates on its public policy environment.

    The Health Center's strategymakers must be concerned about their ability both to analyze and influence the center's public policy environment because the relationships between numerous public policies and this organization are direct. For example, the center sees its revenues, markets, and the technologies it uses directly affected by public policies. Furthermore, its activities in pursuit of the education, research, and patient care components of its mission are directly affected by public policies.

    As is discussed in Chapter 4, perhaps the clearest way to visualize the depth and magnitude of the relationship between what goes on in a healthcare organization's public policy environment and its organizational performance is to recognize that the ultimate performance outcomes achieved by the organization—whether measured in terms of financial strength, reputation, growth, quality, competitive position, services provided, or other parameters—begin with and are heavily influenced by the nature of the opportunities and threats provided by or imposed on the organization from its external environment. Figure 4.1 illustrates that public policies, along with the other variables in the center's external environment, provide it with a set of opportunities and threats to which its strategymakers must respond.

    In view of this, the Health Center's strategymakers, like those in other healthcare organizations, have developed operational commitments both to analyzing the effect that public policies have on the center and to influencing the policies that affect the center. These operational commitments recognize their dual responsibilities of analyzing and influencing the center's public policy environment to the center's strategic advantage.

3. *How are the Health Center's strategymakers organized to carry out their responsibilities for analyzing and influencing the center's public policy environment?*

As is discussed in Chapter 4, strategymakers in large and complex healthcare organizations usually build into their organizations' structures some formal means of accomplishing the environmental analysis function, although their designs for this do tend to be rather idiosyncratic. Frequently, the designs build the activities associated with analyzing public policy environments into the larger workloads of units that are designed to conduct generic environmental analyses, often in units or departments that also are responsible for overall strategic planning or public affairs. It must be remembered, however, that strategymakers cannot assign their responsibility for this activity to any department or unit. They can only seek through such organizational units to have support and assistance carrying out their responsibility in this area.

As is discussed in Chapter 5, the activities involved in influencing public policy environments are typically not assigned to separate departments or units, in contrast to the way organizations typically handle the assignment of activities associated with analyzing public policy environments. There are exceptions to this, of course, especially so in the largest and most complex of these organizations. When organizations do establish departments or units that are specifically charged to conduct work related to influencing their public policy environments, the departments are usually called public affairs departments or government affairs or relations departments. Some very large organizations even divide the activities into separate departments or units for the federal government and for the state government.

The Health Center has chosen not to organize either the analyzing or influencing activities exclusively into particular departments or units. Instead, the work is highly decentralized and spread through a number of units as can be seen in Figure 7.1. The director of information services, to whom the News and Information Department reports, is heavily involved in activities that are related to analyzing and influencing the center's public policy environment. The associate director for fiscal affairs, to whom both the Data Analysis Department and the Budget Office reports, is also heavily involved, especially in the analysis activity.

Regarding the parts of the public policy environment that affect research funding and activities, the associate director for research and the sponsored programs administrator are involved. They will, for example, closely follow congressional policies that affect the NIH. Regarding those environmental aspects that are crucial to the center's educational mission, the associate director for medical education plays an important role in both environmental analysis and influence. These members of the Health Center's staff will, for example, be especially interested in Medicare policies as they pertain to payment for teaching activities and in policy-relevant activities at the HCFA, where the rules to implement Medicare reimbursement policy are established. The chief of staff and the associate director for patient services are more involved with the public policy issues that directly affect patient care. They might also be interested in Medicare reimbursement policy, for example, but more in terms of how it affects patient care. They also will be interested in Medicaid policies because they are so important to revenues for patient care.

As is discussed in Chapter 5, when an organization widely spreads the work of supporting efforts to analyze and influence its public policy environment effectively, coordination of this work becomes crucial. This certainly is the case at the Health Center where this support work is highly decentralized and diffused within the organization. The most important way to ensure the effective coordination of the analysis and influence work is for the strategymakers in the Health Center, especially the director, to insist that the coordination occur. The director, along with the other strategymakers at the center can by their ultimate responsibility for, authority over, and by their involvement in these activities see to it that expertise and insight held by a variety of people on the center's staff is effectively coordinated and that it supports the overall effort to analyze and influence the center's public policy environment.

However, as is also discussed in Chapter 5, the challenges involved in the dual efforts of strategymakers in healthcare organizations to analyze and correctly interpret the effect of relevant issues in their public policy environments and to influence these environments to the strategic advantage of their organization are quite substantial. Not in the least because so many others, including strategymakers in other healthcare organizations, are simultaneously seeking to exert their own influence in pursuit of their own preferences in these environments. Strategymakers at the University of Texas Health Center at Tyler, cannot hope to meet these challenges successfully by relying exclusively on the use of their own internal resources. Indeed, the center's strategymakers, like those in all healthcare organizations, must frequently turn for assistance to outside resources in fulfilling both their analysis and influence responsibilities.

The primary source of outside assistance, as was noted in the discussion accompanying Question 1, is the interest groups to which strategymakers and their organizations belong. The Health Center can rely upon its membership in the AHA and in the COTH for assistance. The center's strategymakers can also rely upon help from the Board of Regents and the Office of the Chancellor of the University of Texas System, especially in dealing with the state level of their public policy environment.

4. *How should the strategymakers at the Health Center analyze its public policy environment?*

As is discussed in Chapters 2 and 4, the analyses of public policy environments for healthcare organizations are only parts of larger situational analyses, which are themselves parts of a still larger strategic management process in these organizations. It may be useful to go back to Chapter 2 and review Figure 2.1.

The focus here is restricted to the external analysis of the public policy environment of the Health Center. When properly conducted, such an analysis unfolds in five related steps:

- environmental scanning to identify strategic public policy issues (i.e., specific public policies as well as the problems, possible solutions to the problems, and political circumstances that might eventually lead to actual decisions that could affect the organization);
- monitoring the strategic public policy issues identified;
- forecasting or projecting the future directions of strategic public policy issues;
- assessing the implications of the strategic public policy issues for the organization; and
- diffusing the results of the analysis of the public policy environment among those in the organization who can help formulate and implement its strategies.

5. *What strategic public policy issues face the Health Center?*

As is discussed in Chapter 1, public policies that pertain directly to healthcare organizations or that are strategically relevant to them constitute a very large set of decisions. Some of these decisions are codified in the statutory language of specific pieces of legislation. Others are the rules and regulations established to implement legislation or to operate government and its various programs. Still others are the judicial branch's relevant decisions. Furthermore, as is discussed in Chapter 4, the large set of public policies that are of strategic importance to healthcare organizations such as the Health Center represent only part of what must be considered strategic public policy issues. The problems, potential solutions to the problems, and political circumstances that might align to lead to policies must also be considered important strategic public policy issues. These, too, must be taken into account in a complete analysis of the center's public policy environment. Thus, effective scanning of the Health Center's public policy environment involves identifying not only specific policies that are of strategic importance to the organization, but also identifying emerging problems, possible solutions to them, and the political circumstances that surround them that could eventually lead to modification of these policies or to new policies.

There are direct and powerful links between public policies, at both federal and state levels, and the strategic decisions that guide, shape, and direct healthcare organizations. This is certainly the case at the Health Center. Examples of some of the public policies that are strategically important to the center are:

- Medicare and Medicaid reimbursement policies, because the center receives more than half of its patient care revenues from these sources.
- Federal policies affecting the NIH, especially its funding, because the center conducts research with grants obtained from the NIH.
- The Texas Legislature's appropriations policy, because the center relies upon this source of funds to offset some of its costs of caring for indigent patients.
- Regulatory policies of the FDA, because the center seeks to develop new medical technology through its research activities.
- Operational regulations imposed on the center by the state of Texas and by the University of Texas System, because these entities prescribe the center's mission (i.e., education, research, and patient care).
- Federal and state policies regarding graduate medical education, because the center operates a family practice residency program.
- Federal and state policies pertaining to employees (i.e., licensure of personnel, scope of practice, fair labor practices, and support for educational programs for health professionals, among others), because the center employs a workforce of over 1,300 people.
- State regulations pertaining to facility licensure, because the center operates as a healthcare facility in the state of Texas.

As a means of emphasizing the strategic importance of these public policies to the Health Center, consider for example (as is done in Chapter 1 for healthcare organizations in general) the extraordinary effects on its strategic decisions the policy changes that have been under consideration for the Medicare and Medicaid programs in recent years would have on the center. Its strategymakers have had to consider such strategic questions as these:

- How would reductions in Medicare and Medicaid reimbursement rates affect the Health Center's strategies?

- If changes in Medicare and Medicaid policies reduced the volume of activity, how would this be handled? What staff reductions might be needed, and how would they be handled?
- What proportions of the Medicaid and Medicare populations that the Health Center serves could be enrolled in managed care programs in the future? What would the effects of such changes be on the Health Center?
- How much and at what rate are inpatient use rates for Medicaid and Medicare clients expected to change? How will the Health Center adjust to these changes?
- What policy changes is the state of Texas likely to make in view of efforts by the federal government to shift more of the costs of the Medicaid program to the states? How will the possible policy changes Texas makes affect the Health Center?

6. *How should the Health Center's strategymakers seek to influence the center's public policy environment?*

As is discussed in Chapter 5, the exertion of influence in public policy environments is a process through which people successfully persuade others to make decisions or take actions that they want them to make or to take. But, as is also discussed in Chapter 5, to have influence one must also have power. This is so because power, in the context of market relationships and exchanges, whether the exchanges occur in economic or political markets, is the potential to exert influence. More power means more potential to influence others. Therefore, as is noted in Chapter 5, if one is to understand influence, one must first understand and be able to acquire and use power. But how do they obtain power? What are the various sources of power available to them?

The strategymakers at the Health Center—indeed, strategymakers in all healthcare organizations—have three bases of power that permit them to have influence in their organization's public policy environment:

- positional power, which is derived from a person's position in a social structure or in an organization; this form of power is also called formal power or authority. It exists because societies find it advantageous to assign certain powers to individuals in order for them to perform their jobs effectively. Thus, elected officials, appointed executives, and judges, as well as strategymakers in healthcare organizations, association professionals, corporation executives, union leaders, individual voters, and many other participants in the political marketplace, possess certain legitimate power that accompanies their social or organizational positions;

- power to reward or coerce others, which is based on a person's ability to reward compliance with (or to punish noncompliance with) the preferred decisions, actions, and behaviors that are sought from others. This form of power stems in part from the positional power a person holds; superiors in organizations have this base of power over their subordinates, leaders in the Congress have it over the members. Such power stems from the ability to supply or withhold from any person one wishes to influence something of value to that person, whether money, vacations, promises of future employment for the person or their family members, and so on; and

- expert power, which is derived from possessing expertise or information that is valued by others. Within the political marketplace, such expertise as that necessary for solving problems or performing crucial tasks can be extremely important.

Importantly, as is also discussed in Chapter 5, these three bases of power in the political marketplace are interdependent. They can and do complement each other. People whose positions in society or in organizations permit them to use reward power, and who do so wisely, can strengthen their positional power. Similarly, people in positions of power typically have more opportunities to either reward or coerce others. Expertise, especially that based on exclusive access to information, is frequently a function of a person's position or access to people in certain positions. Such access can be facilitated through the power to reward or coerce.

Effective participants in the marketplace for policies, those who succeed at translating their power into influence, tend to be aware of the sources of their power and to act accordingly. What distinguishes the ability of certain people to use effectively the power to which they have access—that is, to translate power into influence in the political marketplace—are their interpersonal and political skills.

Having the power to influence a public policy environment, no matter what the base of that power, is only part of the influence equation, however. Strategymakers who seek to exert influence in their organization's public policy environment must know where to focus their attention and efforts. As is discussed in Chapter 5, they should be guided in their efforts to influence policies by identifying public policy issues that are of strategic importance to their organizations (see the discussion of Question 5 above). By focusing in this way, strategymakers will seek to influence strategically relevant policymakers at the federal, state, and local levels of government. Furthermore, they will extend their efforts to influence to those who have influence with these policymakers.

As is noted in Chapter 5, if strategymakers are to influence the policymaking process effectively, in addition to influencing policymakers directly, they must also concern themselves with helping to shape the conceptualizations of problems, the development of potential solutions to the problems, as well as with the political circumstances that help drive the policymaking process. The suppliers of public policies, and those who can influence them, form the appropriate focus for strategymakers who seek to influence the public policies that will affect their organizations. In short, strategymakers must seek to exert their influence throughout the public policy environment of their organization.

In Chapter 5, it is recommended that strategymakers use the model of the public policymaking process, which is shown in Figure 3.1 and replicated in Figure 5.1, as a "map" to help them to identify the places in the process where they can exert influence. This map locates places in the three phases of the policymaking process where attention can be usefully focused:

- policy formulation, which incorporates activities associated with agenda setting (problem definition, identifying solutions, and affecting the political circumstances surrounding the issue) and subsequently with the development of legislation;
- policy implementation, which incorporates activities associated with rulemaking and policy operation; and
- policy modification, which exists because perfection cannot be achieved in the other phases and because policies are established and exist in a dynamic world where events and circumstances routinely render existing policies inadequate and provide new opportunities for those affected by policies to seek to help change them.

In Chapter 5, a consideration of the sources of power that strategymakers have (power based on position, power based on the ability to reward and coerce, and power based on expertise) is combined with a consideration of the various places in the policymaking process where influence can be effectively exerted to form a grid that is shown originally in Figure 5.2 and replicated below as Figure 7.2, with the modification of labeling the cells.

The cells in this grid, each identified by a letter, represent the specific combinations of *where* in the public policymaking process influence can be exerted and the *sources* of the influence that can be exerted in each place. An appreciation of the sources of the power to exert influence is the starting point for considering how influence can be effectively exerted. In effect, this grid can serve as stimulus for strategymakers to think about where and how they might exert influence in the public policymaking

Figure 7.2   The Opportunities to Exert Influence in Public Policy Environments

	Problem Definition	Identifying Solutions	Political Circumstances	Legislation Development	Rulemaking	Policy Operation
Power Based on Position	cell (a)	(b)	(c)	(d)	(e)	(f)
Power to Reward/Coerce	(g)	(h)	(i)	(j)	(k)	(l)
Power Based on Expertise	(m)	(n)	(o)	(p)	(q)	(r)

process. Some hypothetical examples drawn from the context of the University of Texas Health Center at Tyler are illustrative.

In cell (a), the center's strategymakers would focus on the ways their positional power could be used to help define and document problems that could be addressed through public policy. For example, as strategymakers in a state health center they are positioned to help policymakers understand the magnitude of the problem of the lack of health insurance among Texans. These strategymakers are in a position to document the extent and some of the implications of the problems for policymakers. Furthermore, their positions as strategymakers of a healthcare organization—that is, as occupants of its strategic apex—permit them to call on others for assistance in this effort. Obviously, they can call on other members of the staff at the Health Center. They can also solicit the help of their strategymaking counterparts in other healthcare organizations in the state to buttress their documentation of the problem. They can even call on interest groups to which they belong, such as the Texas Hospital Association, to help in this process.

In cell (j), the Health Center's strategymakers would focus on the ways in which their ability to reward or to coerce policymakers could be used to exert influence in the development of specific legislation that would be to the center's strategic advantage. Although the case does not specifically address the issue, it might well have been that the center's strategymakers had this source of influence with the state senator from Tyler who introduced the 1977 legislation that transferred control of the Health Center to the University of Texas System. The rewards could have been the obvious ones, such as campaign support, but they could also have been in the more intangible form of working with the senator to permit and facilitate the accomplishment of something that was extremely important to the future of the senator's district in terms of its economy and its healthcare services, as well as being of strategic advantage to an important organization within his district.

In cell (n), the center's strategymakers would focus on their opportunities to use the power to exert influence that derives from expertise to help identify and implement policy solutions to problems. For example, when the Texas Legislature granted $1 million to the Health Center in 1993 to establish and operate the Center for Pulmonary Infectious Disease Control it did so in response to the Health Center's development of a proposal for the new center—a proposal that reflected the Health Center's considerable expertise in this area—as an important step in the fight against the resurgence of tuberculosis in the state.

In cell (q), the Health Center's strategymakers would focus on their opportunities to use expertise within the center's staff to influence the final wording on rules and regulations that affect the center's organizational performance. For example, there is expertise within the center's staff that would be relevant to the promulgation of rules pertaining to funding and operation of graduate medical education programs such as the family practice residency; Medicare reimbursement formulae and practices; and the award of NIH research grants, as well as in many other areas. It is a routine matter for strategymakers at the center, as is the case with strategymakers from similar organizations, to use their expertise as a mechanism to influence the formulation and implementation of rules that affect their orgnization.

In cell (c), the center's strategymakers would think of ways in which their power to influence based on position could be used to change political circumstances surrounding an issue. For example, the members of the board of regents, who are part of the Health Center's strategic apex by virtue of their board positions, can and do exert influence on the members of the Texas Legislature. This influence helps determine the state's funding for the University of Texas System, including the center's state funding.

The examples given above are not exhaustive. Each of the cells that is discussed contains many other examples of the nexus where influence can be exerted and how it can be achieved. And, for several of the cells—such as cells (e), (f), (h), and (k)—no examples are given. The examples are intended only to stimulate the readers to think about the possibilities in this grid. It should be noted, in this regard, that the real world is not fully captured by this model. By suggesting that the cells can be thought about one at the time, the model is an oversimplification of reality. More realistically, strategymakers operate in several cells simultaneously even when they are trying to influence a single policy issue. Moreover, they typically focus on many issues at any point in time.

This complicates things considerably. However, this grid does illustrate a very important point for strategymakers. They have many places in the policymaking process where their influence can be legitimately and effectively exerted, and they have more than one source of influence in each of these places.

7. *What ethical considerations should the Health Center's strategymakers take into account in their efforts to influence the center's public policy environment?*

As is discussed in Chapter 5, ethical behavior for strategymakers who seek to influence policy can be guided in important ways by four philosophical principles: respect for the autonomy of other people, justice, beneficence, and nonmaleficence.

The principle of respect for autonomy is based on the notion that individuals have the right to their own beliefs and values and to the decisions and choices that further these beliefs and values. This principle includes several other elements that are especially important in guiding ethical behavior in those who seek to influence policymaking. One of these is truth telling. Respect for people as autonomous beings implies honesty in relationships with them. Closely related to honesty in such relationships is the element of confidentiality. Confidences broken in the policymaking process can impair the process. A third element of the autonomy principle with relevance to the policymaking process is fidelity. This means doing one's duty and keeping one's word. When strategymakers who seek to influence policy tell the truth, honor confidences, and keep promises, their behavior is more ethically sound than if these things are not done.

Justice is a second ethical principle of significant importance to those who seek to influence policymaking. The practical implications for public policymaking of the principle of justice are felt mostly in terms of distributive justice; that is, in terms of fairness in the distribution of healthcare benefits and burdens in society. The center's service to uninsured people, and their efforts to have the state fund these activities, reflect adherence to the principle of justice. Attention to the ethical principle of justice, of course, raises the question of what is fair. Allocative policies that adhere closely to the principle of justice allocate burdens and benefits according to the provisions of a morally defensible system rather than through arbitrary or capricious decisions. Regulatory policies guided by the principle of justice, such as those that govern the center's state license, affect fairly and equitably those to whom the regulations are targeted.

Two other ethical principles have direct relevance to policymaking and to efforts by strategymakers to influence this process: beneficence and nonmaleficence. Beneficence in policymaking means acting with charity and kindness. This principle is incorporated into acts through which benefits are provided, thus beneficence characterizes most allocative policies. But beneficence also includes the more complex concept of balancing benefits and harms, for using the relative costs and benefits of alternative decisions and actions as one basis upon which to choose from among alternatives. The growing emphasis on cost-effectiveness in healthcare and the development of policies to achieve this goal will increasingly call into play the principle of beneficence in developing ethically sound policies. Strategymakers at the Center, as well as those in other healthcare organizations, would be in danger of violating this principle of ethical behavior should they seek policies that exclusively serve the interests of their organization rather than maximizing the net benefits to society as a whole.

Nonmaleficence, a principle with deep roots in medical ethics, is exemplified in the dictum *primum non nocere*—first, do no harm. When strategymakers who seek to influence policy are guided by this principle, they seek to minimize harm to society as a whole. The principles of beneficence and nonmaleficence are clearly reflected in health policies that ensure the quality of healthcare services and products. Such policies as those establishing PROs to review the quality of care provided to Medicare patients and the policies that the FDA uses to ensure the safety of pharmaceuticals are examples. Policies that support the conduct and use of outcome studies of clinical care are also examples.

Although adherence to the principles of respect for the autonomy of other people, justice, beneficence, and nonmaleficence does not ensure that policies supported by strategymakers necessarily are in the best strategic interests of their organizations, such adherence does place the strategymakers on relatively high ethical ground. This is the appropriate place for strategymakers to be.

8

Conclusion

I noted in the Preface the possibility that strategymakers in contemporary American healthcare organizations may be operating under a curse—one to the effect that they must live in "interesting times." No one knows for certain about the curse, but there is no doubt that these are interesting times for the strategymakers. Nor is it likely that the times will be any less interesting in the foreseeable future.

One of the more volatile and important aspects of the times for healthcare strategymakers is the public policy environments that their organizations face. The purpose of this book has been to help the reader better understand these environments and the link between them and effective strategymaking. Specifically, I have pointed out that strategymakers have dual responsibilities regarding their organization's public policy environment. On the one hand, they should be adept at *analyzing* this environment and at factoring the information thus obtained into their strategymaking. On the other hand, they should be adept at *influencing* their organization's public policy environment to the strategic advantage of their organization. Fulfilling these responsibilities fully and ethically will lead to remarkable rewards: better strategymaking in healthcare organizations and better public policymaking to guide the nation's pursuit of health.

Index

About the Author

Beaufort B. Longest, Jr., Ph.D., is Professor of Health Services Administration in the Graduate School of Public Health, Professor of Business Administration in the Katz Graduate School of Business, and the founding Director of the Health Policy Institute at the University of Pittsburgh. Previously, he was on the faculties of Georgia State University and of the Kellogg Graduate School of Management at Northwestern University. A Fellow of the American College of Healthcare Executives, his research on issues of health management and policy has received substantial external funding support and has resulted in numerous publications. He is co-author of *Managing Health Services Organizations*, Third Edition, one of the most widely used textbooks in graduate health management programs, and is the author of *Health Policymaking in the United States*, which is also widely used as a textbook. His most recent book, published in 1996, is *Health Professionals in Management*. He consults widely with associations, government agencies, healthcare organizations, and universities on health policy and management issues.